Diane Richardson is well-known around the world for her work on safer sex and how AIDS affects women. The author of the highly acclaimed book, *Women and the AIDS Crisis* (also published by Pandora), she teaches sociology at the University of Sheffield, and recently she was Visiting Fellow at Murdoch University, Perth, Western Australia.

SAFER SEX

THE GUIDE FOR WOMEN TODAY

DIANE RICHARDSON

PHOTOGRAPHS BY
LESLEY THOMSON

CARTOONS BY
ROS ASQUITH

LONDON SYDNEY WELLINGTON

First published by Pandora Press, an imprint of Unwin
Hyman Ltd, in 1990.

Pandora Press
UNWIN HYMAN LIMITED
15–17 Broadwick Street
London, W1V 1FP

Allen & Unwin Australia Pty Ltd
8 Napier Street, North Sydney, NSW 2060, Australia

Allen & Unwin New Zealand Pty Ltd with the
Port Nicholson Press
Compulsales Building, 75 Ghuznee Street, Wellington,
New Zealand

British Library Cataloguing in Publication Data
Richardson, Diane
    Safer sex: the guide for women today.
1. Women. Sex.
    I. Title
    612'.62

    ISBN 0–04–440490–5

Designed by Liz Black

Typeset by Wyvern Typesetting Ltd, Bristol

CONTENTS

ACKNOWLEDGEMENTS

Now that this book is finished I want to thank all the people who, in different ways, have helped me along the way. Firstly thanks to Candida Lacey, my editor, for her helpful comments and support when I needed it. I also want to thank Ginny Iliff at Pandora Press. My additional thanks to Debby Klein and Doreen Massey for reading and making comments on the manuscript. I also want to thank my friend Jean Carabine for her helpful comments. Thanks also to Liz Trinder for rescuing me whenever the computer and I did not get along, and to Tracy Nathan and Carol Webster for their help and interest.

Various people and organisations provided information and advice and I would like to thank them, in particular workers at the Terrence Higgins Trust, the Family Planning Association, the Health Education Authority and CLASH. I also owe a very special thanks to all the women I spoke to who were willing to share their experiences, and whose comments I have used, and to the people who gave of their time and interest in being photographed for this book.

Writing a book, though a challenging and at times an exciting experience, is not good for your social life. Too often it has prevented me from spending time with the people I love and have fun with. Yet my friends have continued to provide me with a great deal of emotional and practical support, as well as putting up with me going on endlessly (yet again) about sex. Thanks Ann, Jackie, Mary, Jean, Liz and, especially, Libby.

Sheffield
January 1990

Lesley Thomson wishes to acknowledge her father Bill Thomson, who taught her to take photographs, and the cabaret act Parker & Klein for their inspiration and support.

INTRODUCTION

There are lots of books about sexuality, but there are still very few that are based on what women experience and might want from a sexual relationship. Also, in the last few years, with the emergence of AIDS, our ideas about sexuality have begun to change. These are good reasons for wanting to write a book about safer sex for women. But they are not the only reasons. Safer sex is itself about looking at our sexuality and relationships in new and different ways.

Most books talk about sex as if it were similar to learning to ride a bicycle or play tennis; a matter of learning the right technique. We know that, in real life, sex just isn't like that. It's not simply a matter of pressing the right button and away we go. Sexual learning is much more complicated than memorizing an instruction manual. It has to do with how you feel about your body and how much you know about how it works. It has to do with how you relate to others, and emotions like love, passion, friendship, tenderness and desire. It also involves issues about power and control in relationships.

Very often discussions about safer sex ignore these things. They tend to assume that all people need are the facts about what is considered to be safe, or safer, sexual practice, and what comes into the 'high-risk' category. Very often facts are not enough. We need ways to help us feel more assertive and say what *we* expect and want from sex. That's why this book discusses not only how to reduce risk of pregnancy, AIDS or other sexually transmitted diseases, but also how to negotiate safer sex.

This book is meant for women, but that doesn't mean that safer sex means the same thing to each of us. One woman may be concerned with preventing pregnancy, another may think about safety more in terms of reducing the risk of sexually transmitted diseases and AIDS. In some cases it may be about a woman protecting herself from physical and emotional abuse from a partner. It provides you with information to help *you* to decide what safer sex means to you and what changes, if any, you want to make in your relationships. Here is an opportunity to think about the kind of sex you want, as well as how you can enjoy sex safely.

Safer sex needn't mean no more fun or excitement. On the contrary, you may find that as well as being good for your health, practising safer sex helps you to learn more about your body and discover what you really enjoy and find satisfying.

CHAPTER ONE

FEELING
GOOD
ABOUT OURSELVES

Most women find it easy to come up with a long list of things they don't like about their bodies. It is usually more difficult to identify those parts of the body we feel *good* about.

This is not surprising. As children, we are discouraged from exploring or touching our bodies, especially 'down there', and we are taught that our bodies are really there to please others rather than ourselves. Even the language we use to describe women's bodies frequently conveys a negative message; to call someone a cunt or a twat, for instance, is a gross insult.

The media's obsession with women's bodies, particularly women's breasts and legs, also shapes our experience and everywhere we go we are surrounded by images of women. Walking down the street we pass by hoardings which are covered with women's bodies, or parts of bodies, selling cars, alcohol, shampoo, cigarettes – you name it. Watching television we are shown women preparing food, washing up, cleaning, and always looking good. Flicking through magazines and newspapers we are presented with advertisements for products to help us get rid of spots, unwanted hair, cellulite, flab, body odours; in between, articles tell us how to make ourselves look more attractive through dress, cosmetics and dieting.

Get your ads off my body

1

Very few of us actually look like the images of women in advertisements, magazines and films. What are these images telling us? The message is: Your body is not good enough! Only when you have made yourself up, plucked your eyebrows, shaved your legs and underarms, deodorized your body and achieved the 'perfect' figure can you expect to be loved and admired. It's no wonder many women dislike their bodies, feeling that they do not live up to what is considered is attractive.

These feelings can affect our self-esteem. Am I too thin, or too fat? Does my breath smell? Is my skin wrinkled? Even though we might feel resentful and angry that women are more frequently judged by how they look rather than by who they are, most of us still worry about a particular aspect of our appearance.

A woman's feelings about her body, whether she likes it or not, will also affect how she thinks and feels about sex. It's hard to relax and enjoy touching and being touched if you are worried about how your body looks, smells or tastes. You might only want to have sex in the dark, you might feel embarrassed about sitting up to make love because you are self-conscious about your tummy and breasts flopping about, or it may be that time of the month, when you feel swollen and flabby. If you are not worrying about your body, and whether your partner is judging you, then it's far easier to enjoy sex. Having a bath with your partner, undressing each other, being massaged, are all things that you can do to get to know each other better and feel more at ease. And for many of us, it's looking at our lovers, smelling and tasting their bodies, that makes sex exciting and enjoyable.

Of course there are many other reasons, besides how we feel about our bodies, why sex can be difficult or embarrassing. You might be worried about becoming pregnant or getting AIDS or some other sexually transmitted disease. It might be a long time since you have had sex with anyone or you might not have had a sexual relationship before. Some of us are shy with other people unless we know them really well, and even then we might feel bashful about making love with a friend or an ex-lover. But feeling good about our bodies can also help us to feel more confident about doing what we enjoy and not doing what we don't like. A woman may find it very difficult to ask her partner to talk to her while making love, to make love without intercourse or to ask for what she wants, because she may be too embarrassed or she may feel insecure about the way her partner feels about her. Does this person really desire me? Do they really want to be doing this with me? Not liking yourself and feeling unattractive or ugly is often the reason for this self-doubt. Yet we find someone sexually attractive *because of* their individuality: we fancy them because of their crooked teeth or their big nose or their sticky-out ears! We enjoy touching and looking at someone's body because it is *their* body. We like their hairy chest or drooping breasts, the veins on their penis or the taste of their vagina. What makes sex exciting is exploring and enjoying each other as we really are.

Often we think about sex as being located in particular parts of the body – the erogenous zones. When these zones, especially our lips, breasts, genitals and buttocks, are touched we are supposed to feel sexually aroused. Many women find that this is an unnecessarily restricted view of sex; after all sexual satisfaction is not simply a matter of pressing the right button and it's perfect. Nor is being a sensitive and responsive lover merely a question of memorizing a book of instructions. Whether we find something exciting or not will depend on what it means to be touched by that person, in that way, in that place, at that time. So when you go for an internal examination and take off your clothes, lie down and a doctor or a nurse touches you, it is extremely unlikely that you feel sexually aroused, but in other circumstances you might.

The whole body is a 'sexual organ'. Sex is not something that is restricted to bottoms and breasts. What happens when the person you've

What feels good?

3

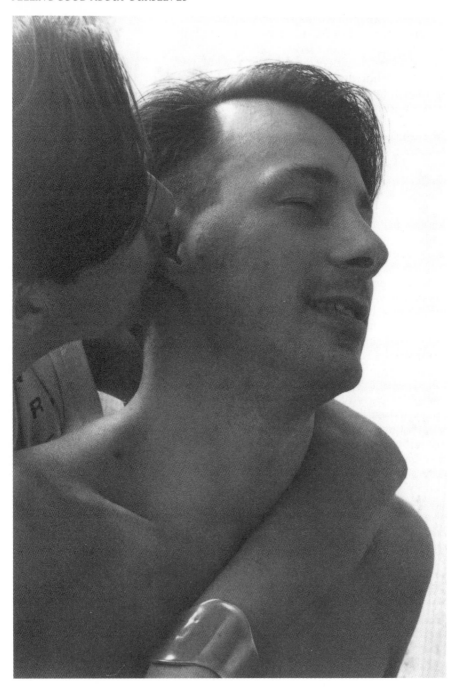

fancied for age brushes past you or accidentally touches your elbow? Don't you feel a shiver of excitement?

Many women are turned on when they are touched on parts of the body which are not usually considered to be erogenous zones – kissing the back of the knee, nibbling an earlobe, slowly stroking the neck and face, licking a palm or sucking fingers and toes, can all be sexually exciting things. Touching fingertips and feeling the skin between the fingers and on the back of the hand can also be very arousing, and so can a back massage or light strokes down the side of the body or the inner thighs.

When you become more aware of your body it's easier to begin to explore ways of touching that make you feel good. Next time you have a bath or are getting undressed, why not spend a little time looking at yourself? Start by asking what do I like most about my body? Don't just focus on one thing – look all over your body, from your fingernails to your toes. Turn around and then to the side. Take a good long look. Concentrate on identifying parts of the body you feel good about. What do you like about them?

When you have come up with a list of at least 10 things about your body that you like, look at those parts of the body that you don't like. Are they really so bad? Think for a minute about why you feel this way? Are they good reasons? Whose standards are you measuring yourself against? Are they standards which most women would find almost impossible to attain? Would you like your friends any less if they looked like this?

It is very common for women to have negative feelings about their breasts, most of us wish they were bigger, smaller, less droopy or just different. We worry about the size and the colour of the nipples and whether they are hairy, or if one breast is a little bigger than the other. After all, when did you last see a Page Three 'pin-up' with small drooping breasts or hairy nipples and stretchmarks?

How well do you know your body?

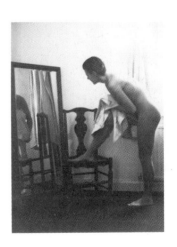

Breasts

5

Adverts and pornography often show women with large breasts as sexy, available playthings for men to look at and comment on. This adds to the barriers which stop us from liking our breasts the way they are. Many women with small breasts feel that they are unattractive and 'unfeminine'. Some are so unhappy that they try to make their breasts bigger by exercising, using pills and lotions or plastic surgery. Women with large breasts, on the other hand, may feel embarrassed, angry or just plain fed up with being stared at and harassed by men.

Clearly, feeling sexually attractive matters to women but that doesn't mean we have to accept stereotypes of what is 'beautiful' or

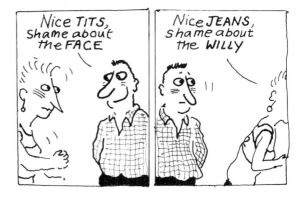

'sexy'. Who's to say that large breasts are any better than small, or drooping breasts any worse than firm? Attractiveness doesn't have to be equated with breasts of a certain size and shape. Most of us find someone attractive because of the kind of person they are, because they make us laugh and feel happy or because we find them interesting – it's not just what they look like. If we can value others the way they are, then why don't we start to do the same for ourselves?

We're all different

Breasts come in all shapes and sizes. Some are large and round, others are small and lemon-shaped. Some are firm to touch, others are soft

6

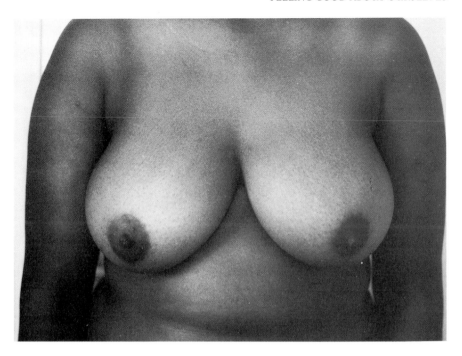

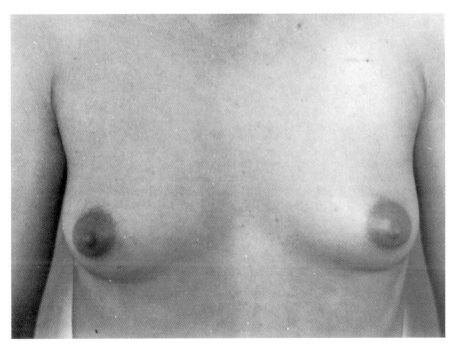

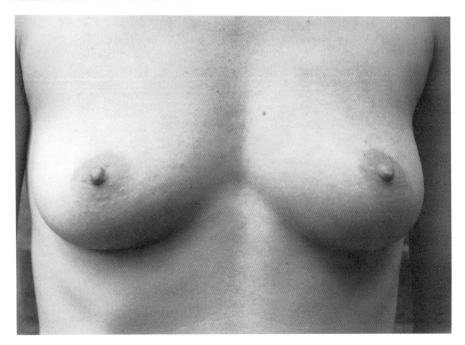

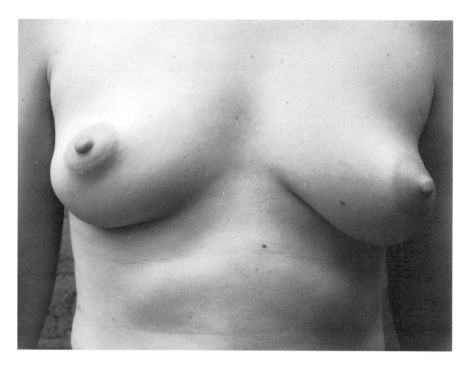

and floppy. Some have scars where perhaps a lump has been removed, or a breast may have been removed altogether. They all differ slightly from each other and the left breast is usually slightly bigger than the right. Each breast contains glands, surrounded by fatty tissue, and it's these glands which produce milk if you have a baby. Nipples, too, vary from woman to woman; some are small and flat and some are like raspberries. Sometimes hair grows around the nipple or in between the breasts, and some women's nipples are inverted, but this doesn't make any difference to the amount of enjoyment you can get from having them kissed or touched.

Nipples are very sensitive to touch and temperature. They get hard and stand out when they are cold or when stroked or sucked. The dark circular area around the nipple, the areola, wrinkles up when the nipple becomes erect and if you look closely you'll see little bumps, called Montgomery's tubercules, in the skin around it. (It may be easier to see these when you are warm and relaxed – perhaps in the bath.) The colour of this part of the breast will be different for every woman. It may be deep brown, black or the palest pink and, as you get older, or if you have a baby, the colour may alter, becoming darker. The size will also vary so that in some women the dark area around the nipples is the size of a small coin and in others it is 3 or 4 times this.

The breasts, nipples and areola change in size when a woman becomes sexually excited. Her nipples harden and become erect, her breasts get bigger as the blood rushes into the veins, and the areola swells too.

Whether your nipples and breasts are large or small makes no difference to how sensitive they are. Sensitivity varies a great deal between women (and in men too). Some women experience very little sensation in their breasts while others become extremely turned on, sometimes to the point of orgasm, when their breasts and nipples are touched, sucked or stroked. It may feel as if there is a direct line of sensation running right through the body, from nipple to clitoris. A woman's breasts may also vary during her menstrual cycle. Some women experience water retention before their period, which can make their breasts feel extremely tender, so that they do not want them to be touched or only lightly and gently. Vitamin B6 tablets in combination with a vitamin B complex, or oil of evening primrose capsules sometimes reduce feelings of bloatedness just before a period, and may make it easier to relax and enjoy making love.

Breast examination It is important for women to examine their breasts regularly because if you do discover a lump, the sooner you have it checked by a doctor the better. Also, by examining your breasts regularly, you will soon get to know what they are normally like so that you are likely to recognise any changes in how they look or feel, and because of the changes during the menstrual cycle it's a good idea to do this at the same time every month. The best time to examine your breasts is just after your period has finished when your breasts are not as full and you are more likely to discover anything unusual. Women who do not have periods should still examine their breasts once a month, too.

Stand in front of a mirror, with your arms relaxed by your side, and look carefully at your breasts. Stretch both your arms above your head and then put your hands on your hips and push down. Look to see whether there are any wrinkles or dimples or bulges in the skin or if there is any change in the nipples since you last examined them. Look for one nipple being unusually withdrawn back into the breast. (Some women are born with inverted nipples, so it's *not necessarily* a sign of cancer.) Do your nipples look asymmetrical, as if they are pointing in different directions? Again, remember that you are looking for *changes* in how your breasts and nipples look. Squeeze each nipple gently to see if there is any discharge coming from it.

Lie down with a folded towel under your left shoulder and your left arm by your side.

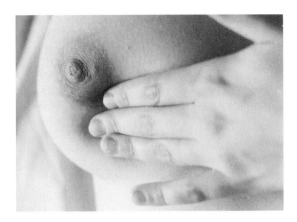

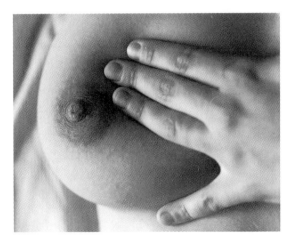

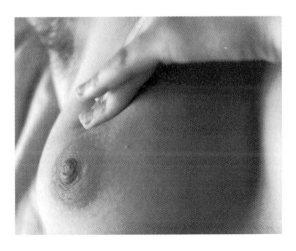

Examine your left breast with your right hand. Feel every part of the breast using the flat part of your fingertips. Move your hand in small circles, pressing down, firmly but softly, until you have covered the entire breast, including the nipple. Raise your left arm behind your head and repeat the whole procedure. Also feel to the side of each breast and under each arm for a lump or thickening of breast tissue. To examine your right breast put a folded towel under your right shoulder and repeat the examination as you did for the left.

Do the same thing, examining each breast thoroughly, sitting or standing. Changing position may allow you to discover a lump that you couldn't feel when you were lying down.

If you do discover anything which seems different from usual, you should go to see your doctor. Don't be afraid of going to see him or her; 9 out of 10 lumps are not cancerous, simply harmless cysts. But it could be cancer and, if it is, the sooner you see a doctor the better your chances are of being successfully treated. Breast cancer is curable, especially if it is discovered early. So don't wait until it's too late!

Breast cancer

Breast cancer is the most common form of cancer in women and the leading cause of death in women aged between 35 to 54. It is usually treated by removing the affected breast, but some doctors now believe that in certain cases removing the lump without removing the entire breast, and the use of radiation therapy, may be just as effective as a mastectomy (breast removal).

This is an important development in terms of what it means to have breast cancer. For many of us, the fear of losing a breast is almost as great as the fear of having cancer. Typically, what we are afraid of is no longer being sexually attractive. Women who are not in a relationship who have a breast removed, may feel that their sex-lives are over, or become anxious about how they will cope when they eventually do meet someone who they want to have sex with. But some women say that this actually helps you to know right from the start what kind of person the new partner is and whether they are worth bothering with. As one woman said: 'You know if they can accept it that they must really like you for yourself and, funnily enough, that has actually made sex a whole lot better for me.'

For women in steady relationships, a common worry after having a breast or a lump removed is, how will my partner react? Will they still find me attractive and want to make love with me? It's understandable that many women feel this way given that we are used to seeing breasts portrayed as symbols of sexuality and femininity. As a result, some women may not want to have sex because they don't feel desirable anymore, and others may still want to make love but find that because they are more self-conscious about their body, they aren't able to enjoy doing certain things. It may be hard making love with the lights on or sitting naked astride a partner; some women may dislike their partner looking at or touching their chest. How important this is will depend on the kinds of sex a woman enjoys most. If, like many women, having your breasts kissed and stroked is a big part of what makes sex exciting and pleasurable, it may be hard to accept that you can still have a good sex-life after breast surgery. A woman with small breasts may feel this just as strongly as a woman with large breasts. It's not the size that's the main consideration, what matters most is how important having breasts is to a woman's view of herself and her sex-life.

How other people respond will also make a big difference to what it means to have a mastectomy. Women need to be reassured that they are still attractive and friends as well as lovers can help in this respect. But it's important to remember that adjusting to losing a breast can take time. It's understandable that women often feel depressed and lacking in self-confidence after having a mastectomy. Everyone needs to recognise this and possibly their own feelings of discomfort and fear, otherwise their attempts to reassure, however well meaning, may appear insensitive.

13

What's 'down there'?

How many women would recognise a photo of their own vulva? It is hardly surprising that some women are unfamiliar with the different parts of their genitals because as children we are not usually encouraged to touch or look at this part of our body. Although this attitude applies to boys as well, it's easier for them to see what's between their legs! To see your clitoris or labia properly you need to look in a mirror.

The words used to describe women's genitals will also affect the way we feel about touching and looking at ourselves 'down there'. The technical term for a woman's genitals is vulva but there are other words, like cunt or fanny, which are often used as insults, and may convey the message that this is an unpleasant or 'dirty' part of the body. Unfortunately, there are very few alternatives. Take the word clitoris, for example, how many different words for this can you think of? What about labia? It's as if through our use of language we're encouraging girls to think about their genitals negatively or as if they don't exist. The clearest example of this is when a woman's genitals are described as just a hole!

If you look at your vulva in a mirror, or touch it with your fingers, you will find that this is a very detailed part of your body. The curved slope at the front, called the mons pubis or pubic mound, is covered in hair. In some women this is thick and bushy, in other women there is just a fine covering through which you can see skin. As we get older, especially after the menopause, most women find that their pubic hair becomes like this. The distribution as well as the amount of hair also varies between women. It may grow down the inside of your legs, inside your buttocks and up towards your belly button.

Hair also grows on the outer lips, or labia majora, which protect the organs underneath. If you part the outer lips, you will see the inside lips, or labia minora. These lips, which are thinner than the outer lips, and smooth, meet just above the clitoris, forming a fold of skin called the clitoral hood. Both the outer and inner lips are sensitive to touch and many

14

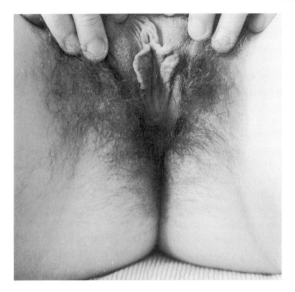

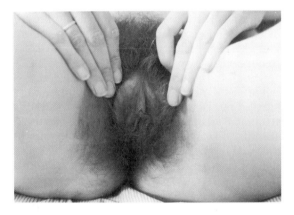

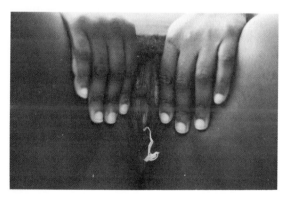

women find stimulation highly arousing. Some women also enjoy touch or pressure on the mons pubis area covered by pubic hair.

Lots of women worry about whether their lips are the 'right' size or shape. This may be because they haven't ever seen another woman's vagina and they aren't aware that in each woman the shape formed by the lips, and the size, is different. There's no 'correct' way! Some women have small, thin labia, others have thick fleshy lips that fold and lap over each other. In many women the inside lips are longer than the outer lips, so that they stick out, and it's not unusual for one of the inner lips to be bigger than the other as well. There is also a great deal of variation in the colour of the labia. The outer lips, which are usually darker than the inner ones, may be a deep reddish brown or chocolate colour. The inner lips may range between soft pink to deep red and mauve, sometimes with shades of pale violet or brown or blue. These colours normally change as we get older, the inner lips becoming a softer rosy-grey.

Something else women worry about is whether their clitoris is too large or abnormally small. The clitoris is the most sensitive part of a woman's genitals and usually it's through stimulation of this organ, either directly or indirectly, that we experience orgasm. Because in the past many books on sex have ignored this part of women's bodies, some women may be unsure about where their clitoris is. In most women the only part that's visible is the tip or glans which looks like a small, shiny pink pearl. Often this is hidden by a fold of skin just beneath the point where the top of the inner lips meet and you may have to gently push this back in order to see it. If you still aren't sure where your clitoris is, try finding it with your fingers. It should feel like a little bump – about the size of a small pea – which is very sensitive when you touch it. But what you can see and touch of your clitoris is only a small part of it; the tip alone can be seen from the outside but inside is a highly sensitive clitoral system of nerves and blood vessels which connect with

16

the vagina and the whole pelvic region.

The size and appearance of the clitoris varies considerably, in some women it pokes out of its hood of skin, whereas in others it is barely visible. This has no bearing on whether you can have an orgasm or not, or how good it feels if you do. The sexual pleasure you can get by stimulating the clitoris has nothing to do with how big it is. Nor is there any truth in the saying that if you masturbate frequently your clitoris will grow bigger – and you won't wear it away either! When you become sexually excited the clitoris swells and becomes engorged with blood. In some women this makes the clitoris become firm and stiff, but not in others. As you become more aroused the area round the clitoris swells up and it may seem as if it disappears but it's just hidden by the lips surrounding it. After orgasm the swelling subsides and the clitoris returns to its usual size and position.

When a woman has an orgasm it always starts in her clitoris, but this doesn't mean that all women like having their clitoris stimulated in the same way. Some enjoy having their clitoris stroked lightly and gently, others find it easier to have an orgasm by fast rubbing movements. Sometimes a woman likes to vary the speed and pressure during lovemaking, perhaps starting off with long, slow strokes before gradually getting faster and firmer. However she likes to be touched, it is always important for her partner to remember that the tip of the clitoris is extremely sensitive to touch and too much pressure can be painful or irritating. Sometimes it feels better when the clitoris is stimulated indirectly by moving the inner lips that surround it up and down, or pressing down on the area just above the clitoral hood.

Between the clitoris and the vagina is an opening, called the urethra, which is where pee comes out. The opening to the vagina is further down towards the point where the inner lips end. In childhood the entrance to the vagina may be partly or totally covered by a thin membrane called the hymen. Some girls worry that this will tear the first time they have sex

clitoral hood

urethra

clitoris

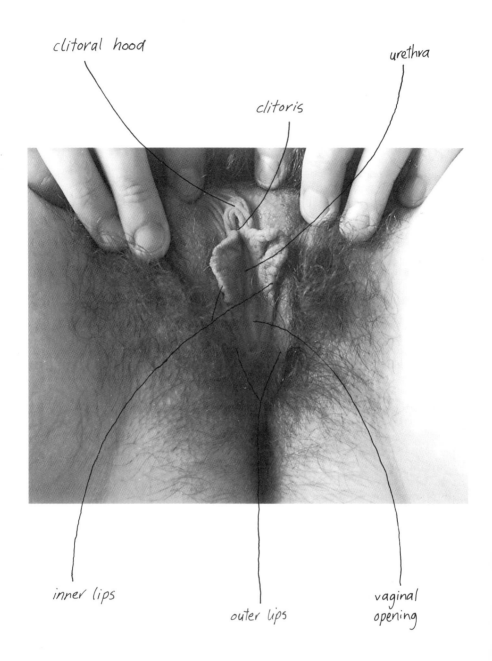

inner lips

outer lips

vaginal
opening

which involves putting fingers or a penis in their vagina, causing pain and bleeding. Most women, in fact, don't notice when their hymen breaks, usually by using tampons or sometimes during sport. When this happens there may be a few spots of blood but it isn't usually painful. And some women are born with only a partial hymen or none at all. You can't necessarily tell if a girl is a virgin by her hymen – another worry some girls may have.

What you see at the entrance to the vagina is not a hole but a fleshy pink opening. If you slide your finger gently inside you can feel that the walls of the vagina are uneven and moist, touching each other. The vagina is a very pliable organ and can change shape and size. When you put a finger or a tampon inside the walls of the vagina can stretch to fit around it. These walls also open out when we are feeling sexually excited, rather like a balloon, as they become thicker and swollen with blood. If you squeeze your muscles as if you were trying to stop yourself from having a pee, you may be able to feel the walls of the vagina tighten around your finger. During orgasm these muscles, called the pelvic floor muscles, contract, and some women find that deliberately contracting and releasing them adds to their sexual enjoyment. Although the vagina can stretch in size to accommodate a finger, tampon or penis, this is not always automatic – it depends on what we are thinking and feeling. If we are relaxed this will be easier. When we are tense or afraid the muscles of the vagina are more likely to contract than expand and this can make it difficult to use a tampon, for example, or to insert a diaphragm or cap. It also means that sex that involves something penetrating the vagina is likely to be quite painful. If you are nervous or scared like this it's important to remember that the kinds of sex women enjoy most don't necessarily involve touching the vagina and so disliking penetrative sex doesn't have to be a problem. You should never feel that you have to do something just because your partner wants to, if you're worried it's going to hurt or you won't enjoy it. If your partner really likes

19

you, they'll want you to feel relaxed and that you enjoy making love.

If you press forward on the front wall of the vagina you may be able to feel a cushion of spongy tissue, about the size of a bean. This is known as the G-spot and it becomes swollen when you are sexually excited. It has been suggested that some women expel a little fluid from the urethra at the time of orgasm as a result of pressure on their G-spot, but it is also argued that this so-called female 'ejaculation' is simply vaginal lubrication or urine. A similar spongy pad between the back of the vaginal wall and the anus also swells and becomes larger when you are aroused. In some women pressure on these areas is exciting but that doesn't mean we should feel we have to go in search of the G-spot, or focus our sexuality on vaginal touch.

Self-examination   Getting to know what your vulva looks like is important for your health as well as your sex-life. If you are familiar with how your vagina normally looks, smells and tastes this can help you recognise when you have an infection.

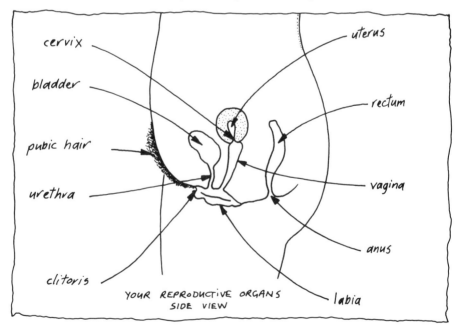

YOUR REPRODUCTIVE ORGANS
SIDE VIEW

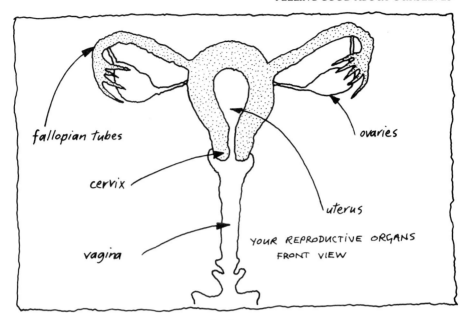

fallopian tubes

ovaries

cervix

uterus

YOUR REPRODUCTIVE ORGANS
FRONT VIEW

vagina

Also, when you know how your body is con-
structed it's easier to start to explore where and
how you like to be touched, and then you will
know when you make love. You can do this by
looking at your genitals in a mirror to see what's
there, and by feeling the different parts with
your fingers. A good time to do this is when
you're feeling warm and relaxed, perhaps after
a bath or lying in bed.

To see inside the vagina you need to spread
the vaginal walls apart using a speculum. This
is a beak-shaped object which you slip into the
vagina and then open out. The cervix looks
different at different times of the menstrual
cycle and some women are able to tell when
they are ovulating or are about to menstruate by
using a speculum. You can see the cervix and
the walls of the vagina better if you shine a torch
onto a mirror so that it reflects the light inside.
Speculums can be bought from chemists and
medical supply firms – the plastic kind are
cheaper and most women find them more
comfortable than metal.

By examining yourself regularly you will
get to know what your vagina and cervix normally look like and will be more able to

recognise signs of infection, rashes, swellings, sores or other problems. Keeping a menstrual chart can also help to identify those changes which are related to the menstrual cycle. Use the one on page 153. If you do notice anything unusual you should check with your doctor.

Although examining ourselves regularly may help us discover vaginal infections, there are some things that it cannot tell us. Unlike breast self-examination, which can help women to detect early signs of breast cancer, it's not possible to tell simply by checking your cervix regularly whether you have any abnormal cells which might progress to cancer, if left untreated. These are easily detected by a cervical smear test. How often you should have the test, what it involves and where you can have it done is discussed on pages 57–9.

Normally the vagina is wet with a clear or slightly whitish fluid, which keeps it moist and clean. The consistency, amount and smell of this vaginal lubrication varies considerably from one woman to another. In some women it may be a thick, copious discharge which smells sharp and musty, others may produce a clear, slippery fluid which smells slightly sweet. It also changes during a woman's menstrual cycle. After a period there may be very little discharge and your vagina may feel dry, then a whitish or cloudy discharge appears which is sticky. Around the time of ovulation this changes to become clear and runnier with a stretchy consistency – rather like eggwhite. It then becomes thick and sticky again. Some women use this knowledge, in conjunction with other bodily changes at ovulation, as a method of contraception. Being familiar with the changes in cervical lubrication can help you predict when ovulation is most likely to occur, and then you can plan your sexual activity accordingly if you don't want to get pregnant. This is sometimes referred to as the cervical mucus or Billings method (see page 40). The thing about this method of birth control is that it cannot damage your health. Alternatively, if you are trying to become pregnant, getting to know the changes in your own body which signal ovulation will help you to plan when intercourse or artificial insemination is most likely to be successful.

Becoming aware of what your vaginal discharge is normally like also makes it easier to recognise when you have an infection because very often discharge smells different and changes colour; and sometimes it feels itchy (vaginal infections are discussed in the following chapter).

When we are sexually excited extra moisture seeps through the walls of the vagina, making our clitoris and vaginal lips slippery and wet. Some women worry that if they don't become wet their partners will think they're not interested in them or in sex. But the fact that a woman doesn't produce much vaginal lubrication doesn't necessarily mean that she isn't aroused and wanting to make love – some women produce very little even when they are extremely turned on. Nor does it necessarily mean that a woman is feeling sexy and about to come just because she is very wet. Health, diet and the time of the month can all affect the amount of vaginal lubrication, as well as its smell and taste. During the menopause and after childbirth it is also quite common for women to experience vaginal dryness. If there is not enough lubrication, rubbing or stroking the clitoris or touching inside the vagina can leave you feeling irritated and sore and as a result, women who are usually dry may sometimes find it hard to relax during lovemaking. But this needn't be a problem. Saliva or a lubricating jelly like KY will make your vulva wet and slippery and more sensitive to touch. (For a discussion of lubricants see Chapter 4.)

If some women worry about being too dry, others worry about being too wet. It may be that they think they'll be seen as raring to go, when maybe they're not, or that they're worried in case their partners think they are 'oversexed', or they may feel self-conscious about being wet because they are afraid they smell. This is why some women dislike the idea of someone stimulating their clitoris, labia and vagina with their mouth and tongue. There are women who don't like touching themselves 'down there' because they feel it is somehow dirty and smelly. Women who are reluctant to touch their genitals may find it difficult to give themselves pleasure by masturbating and, if they need to use contraception, may not feel happy about using a cap or diaphragm. What you use during your period is also likely to depend on how you feel about touching yourself. One of the reasons some women say they prefer Tampax to Lillets is that they don't have to put their fingers in their vagina.

It's not surprising some women feel this way. Adverts for vaginal deodorants encourage us to think of our vaginas as a part of our body that doesn't smell very nice. Vaginal deodorants can cause infections in the vagina and you *don't* need them. Washing with soap and water is all you need to do to keep your genitals clean. And in any case the smell and the taste of a woman's vagina can be very exciting. It's part of what makes oral sex enjoyable and many people really enjoy smelling the scent of their lovers on their fingers after they've made love.

Another anxiety women sometimes have, besides how they smell, is where the vagina goes. For instance, one of the worries some girls have when they first use tampons is that it will disappear inside them and they won't be able to find it again. Others may worry that they will damage themselves putting something of that length in their vagina. The simplest thing to do is to put a finger in your vagina first and feel around. In most women the vagina is about three and a half inches long in a non-aroused state. You may be able to feel the cervix at the end of your vagina (squatting may help you to do this). This should feel a little bit like the tip of your nose, smooth and round, with a small hole or slit in the middle, called the os. If you have had a baby then it will feel more like a chin with a deep dimple in the middle. During your period, the blood flows out from the uterus through the cervix.

Periods   Although menstruation is a normal part of most women's lives, there's still a considerable amount of taboo surrounding it. In the past, and in other cultures, a menstruating woman was often regarded as 'unclean' and capable of strange powers. Nowadays we don't believe that a woman who is menstruating can cause crops to rot or illness and even death, but we still treat her as if it were something to be ashamed of. Even the adverts for tampons and sanitary towels (the term suggests the removal of dirt) emphasize the importance of secrecy.

As well as being something to hide, menstruation is also often seen as a handicap – the time of the month when a woman supposedly becomes incapable of doing certain things and when she is emotionally unstable. Whether it's called 'the curse', 'the monthly blues' or being 'on the rag', having a period is generally referred to in negative terms. Little wonder that some girls feel bad when they first start their periods and are too embarrassed to go into a chemist to buy tampons or pads.

The negative messages we receive about menstruation can also affect our sex-lives. Some women don't want to have sex during their period, especially oral sex, because they feel it's dirty. There's no reason why you shouldn't have sex during a period if you want to (although see page 101 for a discussion on practising safer sex during menstruation). If you are worried about soiling the sheets or getting blood on your partner's fingers, put in a clean tampon. Having a period is nothing to feel ashamed about and hopefully more people are now aware of this. You can buy cards now which congratulate girls on their first period! A far cry from the images we have been presented with in the past.

Menstruation can influence how you feel about sex in other ways. Some women get tense and moody, they have period pains and headaches, and the last thing they feel like doing is making love. (Although some women find it helps to relieve their cramps if they come either by masturbating or making love with someone else.) Others feel bloated and tender and find it difficult to relax and enjoy sex. For some women it's exactly the opposite – they are aroused more easily and feel more sensual just before and during their period. Some women also say that they experience heightened sensitivity around the time of ovulation.

What happens when you have an orgasm?

Although orgasms can feel quite different at different times, your body reacts in a similar way each time you come. When a woman starts to feel excited blood rushes to the genitals, the clitoris increases in size and becomes more sensitive, the outer lips of the vagina become firmer and move apart, while the inner lips go a darker colour and swell and the vagina expands as its walls move apart. It also becomes more lubricated, sometimes making the clitoris and labia slippery and wet. The extra blood also affects the uterus, which is pulled upwards. A woman's nipples usually become firm and erect and her breasts get slightly larger. When the breasts, and especially the nipples, are stimulated the uterus contracts (this is why when a woman goes into labour it may help to keep the contractions going by simulating her nipples). Very often the heartrate and breathing get faster. Some women develop a measles-like rash on their body, usually on the abdomen and chest.

Just before orgasm the inner lips swell even more and change colour, becoming a bright red or deep wine colour. The breasts, nipples and the areola get larger and the inner two-thirds of the vagina opens out like a balloon, while the part near the opening becomes tighter and narrower. In some women the production of vaginal lubrication slows down and they may become dry, especially if this phase lasts a long time.

When you reach an orgasm the muscles surrounding the vagina, uterus and anus contract in a series of short, rhythmical spasms. This usually only last a few seconds, producing intense physical sensations. Often you feel this in your clitoris but you may also feel an orgasm in your vagina or uterus and sometimes the feeling may spread right through your body.

Orgasm is followed by a sense of relaxation

and you may feel tired and drowsy. Gradually the changes that occurred during sexual arousal reverse. Your heartbeat and breathing slow down as you relax, the uterus goes back to its original position, the labia resume their normal colour, the vagina and the clitoris return to their usual size and position, and the swelling in the breasts disappears. If you have been aroused but didn't come, it can take longer for this to happen. Sometimes this produces an aching sensation in the pelvic region due to the continued swelling of tissues with blood.

It can be irritating or even painful to have someone stimulate your clitoris, nipples or vagina immediately after an orgasm but it only usually takes a short time, less than for most men, before a woman is capable of having another orgasm. Some women are capable of having a series of orgasms with only a few seconds in between. Others never experience multiple orgasms but can go on making love for hours and have several orgasms in that time. This doesn't mean that having a series of orgasms is better or more satisfying than having only one. You might have sex and reach orgasm once a week and enjoy it just as much as a woman who has them more frequently. You might never have orgasms and have just as much fun as women who do, orgasm is just one aspect of sexual pleasure. It's not numbers of orgasms which is the important thing for most women, but how they experience them.

Trying to describe an orgasm is difficult because they do not always feel the same. They vary between women and from one situation to the next. Sometimes an orgasm is a warm, tingly feeling which ebbs through your body, while at other times it can be a sharp, shuddering sensation. A lot depends on how you are feeling and what you expect. Books and films often portray orgasm as an ecstatic, earth-shattering experience and it can be like this, but most of the time the earth doesn't move. It is understandable to feel disappointed if your experience of orgasm doesn't live up to expectations but you shouldn't blame yourself or worry that you're

Did the earth move for you?

•

It's hard to say what an orgasm feels like; it varies depending on how I'm feeling and how I'm being touched.

•

27

not 'doing it right'. It's just that we've been misled into thinking that all orgasms should be ecstatic.

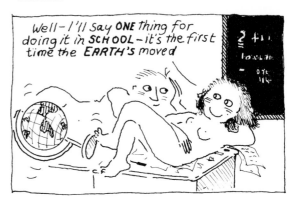

Women sometimes worry about the time it takes them to come. Asking how long it should take to have an orgasm is rather like asking how long a piece of string is. There's no set length; the time it takes will vary depending on who you are with, what you are doing and how you are feeling at the time. Nevertheless the expectation is that women take longer to come than men. As a result, you may feel embarrassed or that you are unusual if you usually come very quickly. This can happen to women who have intercourse with men and come before they do, but lesbians too can be affected by these sexual 'rules'. Other women worry that they are taking too long and that their partner will give up trying or become bored in the process. If you are worried about this, talking about it with your partner may help. You may find that it's not a problem for them or, if it is, that by talking you are able to reassure each other. Making love isn't a race and it shouldn't matter how long it takes.

Sometimes it's like waves of pleasure, at other times it's a short, sharp, shudder of excitement.

For a long time women were thought to have two sorts of orgasms: clitoral orgasm from stimulation of the area around the clitoris and vaginal orgasm from penetration. Vaginal orgasms were somehow regarded as better and more normal than clitoral orgasms – the genuine thing. Nowadays we know that this is not true. All orgasms are clitoral, although a

28

woman can feel an orgasm in her vagina or indeed throughout her whole body. We also know that having something moving up and down in the vagina is not necessarily the easiest way for a woman to come. Many women find it difficult to reach orgasm just through intercourse or by vaginal 'penetration' with fingers, and much prefer to be touched around their clitoris – this is perfectly normal. Even then, an orgasm that comes from rubbing the clitoris may feel very different from one that comes from sucking or licking it.

Where and when you make love will also affect the experience of orgasm. It helps if you are somewhere warm and comfortable and unlikely to be distracted by a knock at the door, the telephone ringing or people bursting into the room. We also experience different sensations when we are wide awake to times when we are feeling sleepy, or irritable. Why you are having sex may also be important. Sometimes it's a way of relaxing or of feeling really close to someone and orgasm is extremely pleasurable. Other times you may have sex when you don't particularly want to, perhaps because it's easier than coping with the hurt look of rejection from a lover, and orgasm is not so fulfilling. Often it's something we do when we're on our own, perhaps when we feel like a good experience, when we're feeling bored or when we are fantasizing about having sex with someone we fancy. Many women find their orgasms are physically much stronger when they masturbate than when they come with a partner, but they may prefer to come with someone else because it is more emotionally satisfying, or because they feel lonely after masturbating.

Most of us have experienced making love without coming. Often it can happen because you're not in the right mood or you have a new partner who is still learning how and where your body likes to be touched. For other women not having an orgasm is normal and they may come only when masturbating. Some women may never have an orgasm. When this happens it certainly doesn't mean that a woman is frigid

●

It's a feeling that starts in my clitoris and spreads out through my body.

●

What can stop us having an orgasm?

or that she can't be aroused and she doesn't enjoy sex. It is probably quite the opposite. Nor does it mean that she's incapable of ever having an orgasm.

There are all sorts of reasons why this can happen. Some conditions, such as diabetes, can sometimes impair orgasm, but in most cases it is how we think and feel about ourselves, our partner and our sexuality that is the key rather than anything physical. Often it's because we haven't been sufficiently aroused or because we are unfamiliar with our body and how it works. We may know what we like but, perhaps because we feel too shy or insecure, we can't communicate this to our partner. A woman may also fail to become sufficiently aroused because her partner is too insensitive and selfish a lover to take the time to find out how and where she likes to be touched. She may feel guilty or embarrassed about enjoying sex if she was brought up to believe that nice girls don't like sex, or that she should never lose control. This is often related to the way women are encouraged to think of sex as something that happens to them rather than something we do for ourselves. Also, they may hold back during sex because they feel that their partner will somehow gain power or control over them, if they come.

Girls are traditionally taught to be careful and not let boys go 'too far'. The message that it is a woman's responsibility to maintain control doesn't make it easy for women to concentrate on themselves and what they want. In order to have an orgasm we need to be able to relax and focus on our feelings, to not worry about pleasing a partner or being on one's guard. This is why some women are able to have orgasms when masturbating while they don't come when making love with someone else – they can forget about anyone else and concentrate on finding out what is pleasurable for them.

It's difficult to get aroused and enjoy sex if you don't feel relaxed. You may be worried about pregnancy or AIDS or you may be scared of getting hurt. One of the problems for some women is that the more they want to have an orgasm, the more self-conscious they become about having one. By trying too hard sex can seem to be a test, instead of just being fun. The important thing is to take pleasure in what you are doing, whether you have an orgasm or not.

When someone asks you 'Did you come?', do you feel you ought to say yes even if you didn't? If you do, it's not surprising. We are encouraged to regard orgasm as the end goal of making love and so we may judge our sexual experiences on that basis. This view of satisfying sex as orgasm can make women feel they're a failure and that they have to pretend that they've come when they haven't. A woman who protects her partner's feelings by faking orgasms may succeed in temporarily massaging an ego, but she's not doing herself or the relationship any favours. For a start, it is usually at the cost of her own pleasure and, as her partner will probably continue doing what they think she enjoys, she may never discover what it takes for her to have an orgasm. If she continues to fake orgasms, she could also begin to hate herself for lying and her partner for not realising. And remember that orgasm isn't what sex is all about for most people – it's just a part of it. There are times when we want an orgasm and times when we are happier making love without feeling we have to come. Sometimes we can have an orgasm but find this less satisfying than when we had sex with someone and didn't come. Knowing our bodies and how they work, feeling that we can tell our lovers how and where we like to be touched, believing that we have just as much right to what we want as they have, are the things that matter if we are to have fun and enjoy sex – whether we have orgasms or not.

Is orgasm what sex is all about?

While for some women not having an orgasm isn't a problem, others feel they would like to explore ways of making this happen. A good place to start is to find out for yourself where and how your body likes to be touched. This is because you can concentrate on what feels good for *you* without feeling inhibited by someone

Learning to have an orgasm

else being there. Some women feel guilty about touching themselves, but why should they? There's nothing wrong with masturbation and most of us do it at some time or other – simply because we enjoy it.

You've got to feel relaxed and in the right mood to have an orgasm. If you are feeling tense and self-conscious about touching yourself, try thinking about things you find a turn on. You might put a record on that you find arousing, or perhaps fantasize about someone you'd like to make love with and what you could do together. Once you are feeling relaxed, start to explore your vulva with your fingers, using different kinds of touch. Do you like it best when you move your fingers lightly over your clitoris or is it more fun when you press harder? Try varying the speed of touch, as well as the pressure. What feels too slow and

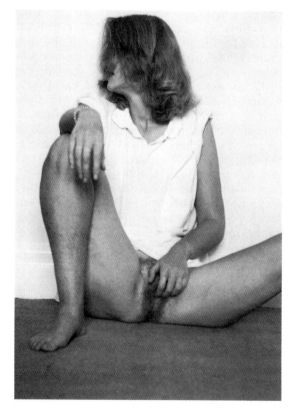

too fast? Move your fingers in different directions and see what difference that makes to the sensations you get. Are there some parts that are more sensitive to certain kinds of touch than others? Is it more exciting to touch the tip of the clitoris or the base? Or perhaps you prefer less direct touch, by moving the lips up and down, or softly touching the area around the clitoris? Move your hands to different parts of your body, using different kinds of touch. You may find that certain areas, and ways of touching, feel more exciting than others. Try touching your breasts and nipples, then go back to your clitoris again. Does it make any difference to how aroused you feel? If your vaginal lips and clitoris are dry, try wetting your fingers with spit or use a lubricant (see pages 132–4 for a discussion of lubricants and the best ones to use). This will reduce friction and help you to discover more easily what kinds of touch you like best. It's important to remember that, like anything else, learning how to come takes time. Don't expect too much too soon. So what if you don't have an orgasm right away, it doesn't mean you can't enjoy yourself.

Some women who have difficulty in having an orgasm have found that by using a vibrator they can come fairly easily. They don't have to be phallic-shaped (you can get them heart and tongue-shaped!) and you may prefer to use a massage set. You needn't worry that you'll become 'hooked' or that you won't be able to come any other way. On the contrary, once you know you can have an orgasm it's often easier to relax and learn other ways of making yourself come. Vibrators and other 'sex-toys' are discussed in more detail in Chapter 3.

If a woman knows how her body likes to be stimulated, it will be easier for her to enjoy sex because she will know what to do to become aroused and can show her partner. Masturbation may also help you to learn to trust your body if you have had a bad sexual experience. The next chapter looks at this and some of the other reasons for developing safer relationships.

CHAPTER TWO

THE
NEED
FOR SAFER SEX

safer sex/ 'saf-er seks/n 1: a way of protecting both partners from the possibility of infection with HIV or other sexually transmitted diseases 2: a way of preventing an unplanned pregnancy 3: taking charge of your life and health 4: being creative and imaginative sexually 5: eroticizing activities you may never have thought could be sexy 6: caring about yourself and your partner 7: protecting yourself from abusive or unwanted sex.

Sex has never been entirely safe, especially for women. But now, with AIDS, we should be all the more aware of the risks involved and the need to practise safer sex. Safer sex includes mutual masturbation, kissing, caressing and stroking, sharing fantasies, licking and rubbing against your partner's body and lots more goodies (see Chapter 3). It isn't just about using a condom! But if your lovemaking is going to include sexual intercourse then always using a condom, plus a spermicide, correctly can make it safer.

Safer sex is about reducing the risk of getting AIDS. It is also about not getting other sexually transmitted diseases, making sure you don't become pregnant unless you want to be, reducing the health risks associated with certain forms of contraception and preventing cervical cancer. We can also think about safer sex in another way. There are all sorts of reasons why sex for women is often unsafe for emotional as well as physical reasons. Women get raped and sexually abused. Women often feel pressurized into having sex just to please their partner. Within some marriages sex may be part of what a man expects of a wife in return for supporting her and any children they might have. When we feel forced into having sex it can shatter our self-esteem. It can leave us feeling

34

exploited and used. Safer sex is about sex we enjoy and feel good about. It's about sex on our terms; sex that reduces the risks to our minds as well as our bodies.

Unplanned pregnancy

There are various ways of preventing an unwanted pregnancy and the safest method is to make love in ways that don't involve intercourse. When you have intercourse and you don't want to be pregnant, you must use a reliable method of contraception and use it well.

What method should I use?

There is no ideal method that's right for everyone. Every method of birth control has its advantages and disadvantages (see pages 42–4). You and your partner have to make a choice by weighing up the pros and cons of different methods to see which suits you the best. Questions you should ask yourself are: How reliable a method is it? What are the risks to my health? Are there any other side-effects? Do I feel safe using it? How will it affect my sex-life? Will it reduce the risk of cervical cancer, AIDS and other sexually transmitted diseases? Would I feel comfortable about using it?

Having explored what you and your partner want from a method of contraception, the next stage is to know what's available and where to get it.

The pill

There are two types of pill: the combined pill and the progestogen-only or 'mini-pill'. The most common is the combined pill which contains two hormones – oestrogen and progestogen – which prevent the release of an egg from the ovaries each month, so that you can't get pregnant. You have to take it every day for 3 weeks and then stop for 7 days, or in some cases 6, when you have your period. If used properly the pill is 99% effective but it may cause side-effects in some women including nausea, headaches, weight gain, bleeding in between periods, water retention, depression, sore breasts and an increased susceptibility to some vaginal infections. If you have any of these side-effects, changing to another brand may be the

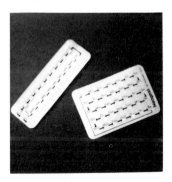

answer. Alternatively, try a different method of contraception. More serious side-effects include high blood pressure, possibly cancer, and more rarely, liver problems and thrombosis. Birth control pills also increase the risk of heart attacks, especially in women who smoke and/or are over 35. Many doctors now advise women who are over 30, and those who smoke, not to use the pill, especially if they've been taking it for some years. If you do stop taking the pill remember that you can get pregnant straight away and so you must use another form of contraception if you have intercourse.

The progestogen-only pill contains only one hormone – progestogen. It is slightly less effective than the combined pill but it has fewer side-effects; while you can be up to 12 hours late in taking the combined pill, you have to remember to take the progestogen-only pill at more or less the same time every day for it to be effective. If you are more than 3 hours late, you may become pregnant.

The morning-after pill is a pill which is prescribed by doctors and which must be taken within 3 days of having unprotected intercourse to prevent pregnancy. It probably works by affecting the lining of the uterus so the fertilized egg is expelled. Although this method is very effective, it is basically an emergency measure.

With injectable contraceptives, such as Depo Provera, progestogen is injected into a muscle and is then slowly released into the body. Each injection lasts for 8 (Noristat) or 12 weeks (Depo Provera), so there is no need to remember to take a pill every day. It works by preventing ovulation and it is very effective, but it can have harmful effects and it is a controversial area of contraception. Some women remain infertile for a long time after they have stopped taking it and, with Depo Provera, there may be an increased risk of cervical cancer.

The intra-uterine device (IUD) or coil

This a small device made out of plastic or copper which is inserted into the uterus by a doctor or a trained nurse. You need to have it

36

changed every 3 to 5 years. IUDs come in various shapes and sizes, with a thread hanging down through the mouth of the cervix to enable you to check that it's still there. You should do this once a week for the first month and then monthly, by inserting a finger inside your vagina and feeling for the thread. If you can't locate it you must go to the doctor or clinic for a check-up. It may be that the IUD has been pushed out without you noticing and you could become pregnant if you have intercourse.

It may increase the length and the heaviness of your periods and some women find it painful to use, if it is fitted badly. The fitting itself can sometimes be painful. As with the mini-pill, you are more at risk of having an ectopic pregnancy (a pregnancy outside the womb – usually in the fallopian tubes) if you do become pregnant while using one. There is also a greater risk of genital infections and pelvic inflammatory disease, and occasionally an IUD may perforate the uterus or cervix.

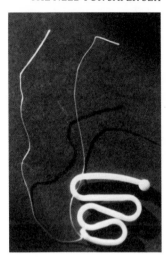

This is a round, shallow dome of thin rubber which fits over the cervix so that sperm cannot enter the uterus. It should ALWAYS be used in combination with a spermicidal cream, foam, film, pessary or jelly so that if any sperm do manage to swim inside the rim of the diaphragm, if it gets dislodged during lovemaking, they will be killed. Using a spermicide that contains nonoxynol-9 will *reduce* your risk of becoming infected with HIV, the virus which causes AIDS (the virus can still get through the vagina walls), as well as getting pregnant (see page 131). Spread the spermicidal cream or jelly carefully. If you make love a second or third time, you should add some new spermicide before having intercourse. After you've finished making love, the diaphragm must be left for at least 6 hours in order to kill the sperm.

The diaphragm

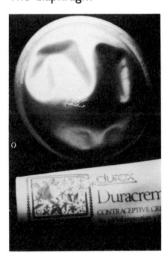

Cervical cap

The cap is a small, thimble-shaped cap which fits over the cervix and is held in place by suction. One advantage of the cap is that it can be worn either for short periods like the diaphragm, or for up to 30 hours. Some women

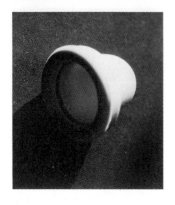

also prefer it to the diaphragm because they can't feel it as much during lovemaking. As with the diaphragm, always use a spermicide.

You will need to be fitted for a diaphragm or cap by a doctor or a nurse, to make sure you get one that is the right size for you and fits properly. Diaphragms range from 55 to 100 mm in diameter; caps are smaller, only 22 to 31 mm in diameter. (You should have it checked every 6 months or if you gain or lose more than 3 kg or 6lbs, after an abortion, miscarriage or the birth of a baby.) The doctor or nurse will also show you how to insert and position it correctly yourself. This can take a little bit of getting used to, so it's a good idea to practise putting it in *before* you use it during intercourse. It is also important to inspect your diaphragm or cap regularly to see if there are any holes which could allow sperm to pass through. Don't use Vaseline or any oil-based lubricant with a cap or diaphragm (hand creams or body lotions, for example), as they dissolve rubber.

Condom

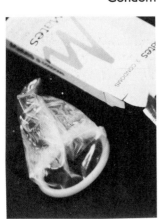

A condom is a thin rubber sheath which fits over a man's penis. This prevents his sperm from entering the vagina during intercourse, as well as preventing sexually transmitted infections, including HIV. Condoms are safe and effective if they are properly used in combination with a spermicide (see pages 112–27). You can get them free from family planning clinics or you can buy them from chemists, supermarkets, garages, toilets and many other places, including mail order catalogues. But remember to check the expiry date on the pack before using them. There are many different types to choose from and so experiment to see which ones you prefer. Some are dry, some are lubricated, they may be smooth or textured, natural or brightly coloured, and some have a reservoir at the tip, others are plain-ended. Most reliable condoms in the UK have a British Standards Kitemark on the pack. Testing is being carried out on a female condom, which is inserted in the vagina (see page 126).

Spermicides

Spermicides are chemical contraceptives which

kill sperm. You can buy different types at the chemist, including jellies, creams, pessaries, film and foams, and in general, foams are more effective than the creams or jellies (see page 131). Spermicides are also available free from family planning clinics. Some women are allergic to the chemicals in certain products, which can cause irritation or soreness, so you should test the spermicide on the side of your wrist before using it for sex. If you do get an allergic reaction, try using a different brand. Again you should also check the expiry date on the pack before use.

Spermicides are not reliable on their own and should only be used as a backup to condoms, a diaphragm or cervical cap – NEVER by themselves. Choose one that contains nonoxynol-9, an active ingredient in many spermicides which may help protect you from infection with HIV and sexually transmitted diseases (see page 131). Leave the spermicide inside your vagina for at least 6 hours after the last act of intercourse, to kill the sperm.

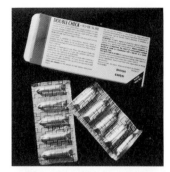

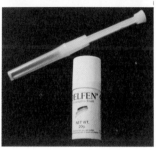

Sponge

This is a soft, mushroom-shaped contraceptive sponge permeated with spermicide containing nonoxynol-9. There is no need to have it fitted – there is one size for everyone. You can buy it over the counter at most chemists. After dampening it with water, to activate the spermicide in the sponge, you insert it into the vagina so that it covers the cervix. The sponge is effective for up to 24 hours, which means that it can be inserted up to 18 hours before intercourse or at the last moment, and again it must be left in place for 6 hours after intercourse. You don't need to add more spermicide if you decide to have intercourse more than once during that time and, unlike most other types of spermicide, the sponge is not messy. Most women also find it comfortable to use and don't notice it once it has been inserted. But, if you have intercourse during your period, you are advised to use another form of spermicide. The sponge is not a reliable method of birth control *on its own* because it is easy to shift out of place during intercourse, but it is a very good

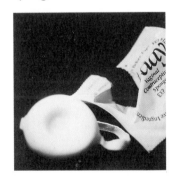

idea to use it in combination with a condom.

Sterilization

In women, sterilization usually involves an operation to block the fallopian tubes to prevent any eggs reaching the sperm. You must be certain in your own mind that you don't want children in future as, in most cases, it is irreversible. If you are under 35 and you haven't yet had any children, it can be difficult to get a doctor to agree to refer you. Sterilization for men is a vasectomy; this is a simple operation where the tubes which carry sperm from the testes to the penis are cut or blocked, so that the sperm cannot enter the semen which is ejaculated when a man comes, but again this needs careful thought.

'Natural' methods or fertility awareness

There are several natural methods of birth control which are based on identifying the time when you are most likely to be fertile. Then you can practise non-penetrative sex, or, if you do have vaginal intercourse during the 'unsafe' days, you could use a condom with a spermicide, but remember that spermicides can make it difficult to interpret cervical mucus signs, so the method becomes less reliable. The temperature method involves taking your temperature every day to pinpoint the time when you are ovulating. After ovulation, your temperature rises slightly. The Billings or mucus method depends on changes in the cervical mucus to indicate when intercourse would be risky. This means examining your cervical secretions. After your period you might get a discharge which is whitish or cloudy and sticky, but just before ovulation this becomes clear and runnier, with a stretchy consistency very similar to eggwhite. Intercourse is thought to be 'safe' 4 days after the clear mucus begins, when the mucus has returned to a cloudy colour. These methods are complicated and you will need to be taught how to recognise the changes in your body which signal fertility. The least reliable of the natural methods is the rhythm or calendar method which involves working out from your previous menstrual cycles a 'safe' period within the current month.

This method is not recommended on its own and it is particularly haphazard if you have irregular periods. Also, as many women discover to their cost, the assumption that ovulation will occur approximately 14 days before the start of the next period is not always correct – a woman may ovulate at any time, including during her period.

What's the safest method of contraception?
The pill and the IUD are the safest ways of making sure you don't get pregnant. Unfortunately, neither of these methods make sex safer when it comes to preventing AIDS and other sexually transmitted diseases and both involve certain health risks. To practise safer sex you should use a condom or make love in ways that don't involve penetrative sex. If used properly, in combination with a spermicide containing nonoxynol-9, condoms are a very good way of preventing pregnancy and sexually transmitted infections. Condoms also help to protect against cervical cancer and they don't pose a risk to your health.

My boyfriend has had a vasectomy. Why do I need to bother with safer sex?
Men who have had a vasectomy may not be able to get you pregnant but they can still pass on HIV and other sexually transmitted infections. To avoid this risk practise safer sex.

I've been on the pill for 5 years now and I'm worried that if I keep on taking it I'm going to increase my chances of getting breast cancer.
Recent research suggests there may be a link between taking the pill and breast cancer, especially for young women who take the pill for a long time. Yet, from other studies, it appears that taking the pill protects against cancer of the ovaries and the uterus.

Contraceptives which need to be fitted or require a prescription, such as the pill, the IUD and the cap, are free from your doctor or from family planning clinics (see page 161 for addresses of clinics). STD clinics will provide

---

You can still get pregnant if:

You are having your period

You douche immediately after you've had intercourse

A man withdraws his penis before he comes

You didn't have an orgasm

You are breastfeeding

You had intercourse just the once

Where to get contraceptives

CONTRACEPTION

THE PILL

ADVANTAGES:

If used correctly, it is extremely reliable

It's easy to take and non-intrusive

It means regular periods

Because it reduces the fear of getting pregnant, sex may be more fun

It protects against ovarian and uterine cancers and pelvic inflammatory disease

DISADVANTAGES:

Remembering to take it every day

There are side-effects and health risks

Some women lose interest in sex

Increased risk of getting some vaginal infections and certain STDs

It doesn't prevent HIV and STDs

THE INTRA-UTERINE DEVICE (IUD)

ADVANTAGES:

Very reliable, especially when used in combination with a spermicide

It doesn't interfere with lovemaking

Once in place it needs checking only occasionally

DISADVANTAGES:

It must be fitted by a doctor or nurse

Side-effects can include painful cramps, bleeding, heavy periods and, occasionally, perforation of the uterus

It can cause pain during intercourse – if it does, it should be removed

It increases susceptibility to infections, especially pelvic inflammatory disease (PID)

It increases risk of STDs, such as chlamydia, spreading to your uterus and ovaries, which can cause infertility

It doesn't prevent HIV or STDs

It may fall out without you knowing – especially early on

If you become pregnant while using an IUD it can cause complications, including miscarriage

THE DIAPHRAGM OR CAP

ADVANTAGES:

It has few side-effects or health risks

You only use it when it is needed

It is very reliable if used properly with a spermicide

Once you've got the hang of it, it's easy to use

It may help to protect against STDs and reduce the risk of cervical cancer

DISADVANTAGES:

It has to be fitted by a doctor or nurse initially

It may interrupt the spontaneity of sex

You need to stop and reapply spermicide if you have intercourse more than once

Some women don't like putting their fingers in their vagina

Your partner may be put off oral sex (cunnilingus) by the taste of the spermicide

It doesn't prevent HIV and STDs

CONDOMS

ADVANTAGES:

They make sex safer than any other form of contraceptive

They will help protect you from the HIV virus and other STDs

They will help protect you from cervical cancer

If used properly in conjunction with a spermicide they are a very effective method of birth control

No health risks

They are free from family planning clinics, easy to buy and simple to use

They can make sex more exciting

Lubricated condoms can make intercourse easier, especially if you are dry

You don't get semen running out afterwards

Flexibility: you only use them when you need to

DISADVANTAGES:

Very occasionally they may cause irritation, burst, tear or slip off

Some people find they interrupt the spontaneity of lovemaking

Some men don't want to wear them

43

SPERMICIDES

ADVANTAGES:

There are no major health risks

They are free from family planning clinics and easy to buy

Some brands help protect you against STDs, including HIV

DISADVANTAGES:

They may cause irritation or soreness

The taste may discourage oral sex

They can be rather messy

You may feel they interrupt the spontaneity of sexual intercourse

Not an efficient contraceptive method if used on their own

They do not protect from HIV and STDs, including HIV

STERILIZATION

ADVANTAGES:

You don't have to worry about becoming pregnant

You don't have to use contraception

It is permanent

Your sex life may be more spontaneous and fun

DISADVANTAGES:

It is almost always irreversible

It offers no protection against HIV infection and other sexually transmitted diseases

There are possible but very rare side-effects and complications

It involves an operation, which many people find difficult and expensive

SPONGE

ADVANTAGES:

You can buy it in most chemists

You don't need to be fitted for one by a doctor or nurse

It gives you 24 hours protection, if you want to have intercourse more than once

It is convenient and simple to use

There is no taste or odour which could put you or your partner off oral sex

It is flexible

There are no major health risks

It isn't as messy as some spermicidal products

DISADVANTAGES:

It can cause a mild irritation of the vagina

It does not totally protect against HIV and other STDs

On its own it is not an efficient method of birth control

FERTILITY AWARENESS

ADVANTAGES:

No cost or health risks

You may feel more in control of your own body

It is non-intrusive

DISADVANTAGES:

There is a risk of getting pregnant

It won't protect you from getting AIDS or any other STDs

It takes time to learn fertility awareness and feel confident with it

It requires the cooperation of your partner

free condoms to men and women or you can buy them in various places: chemists, super-markets, vending machines in pubs, public toilets and garages and by mail order. Spermi-cides are free in family planning clinics and they can also be bought in most chemists – along with the contraceptive sponge.

If you use a reliable method of contraception you can have intercourse with very little risk of getting pregnant, but no method of birth con-trol is 100% safe. You can sometimes tell if you are pregnant soon after conception but you need to wait until your period is 2 weeks late to be sure. If you think you might be pregnant if a condom breaks, there are morning-after birth control methods – either pills or the insertion of an IUD – which can prevent pregnancy (see page 36).

If you do happen to get pregnant and you don't want to be, you will have to decide whether or not to have an abortion. This can be a difficult decision to make, especially if you have been brought up to believe that abortion is wrong. You may find it helpful to talk through how you are feeling with your doctor, someone at a pregnancy advisory service or family plan-ning clinic or a friend. You can get the address of your nearest clinic by looking in the Yellow Pages under Family Planning or Pregnancy Test Services. A good doctor or counsellor will help you to decide without putting pressure on you. Remember, you have a right to choose when and if you should become a mother: it's your body and your life and whatever decision you make it's got to be *yours*.

Abortion

Where can I have an abortion?
Your chances of getting an abortion on the National Health Service will depend on the attitude of your doctor, and where you live. Some doctors don't approve of abortion and will not refer you to a hospital. If your doctor won't refer you, or can't due to long waiting lists, there are various organisations that can arrange for you to have an abortion privately (see page 161). The advantage of this is that it's

usually quicker than an NHS referral and also the other women at the clinic or nursing home will be there for the same reason as you. But it will cost, on average, between £250 and £300. The earlier you have an abortion the safer it is, the easier it is on you and the less it costs.

How is the operation done?

Up to 12 weeks the most common method is by vacuum aspiration or suction. A thin plastic tube is inserted through the cervix and into the uterus. This tube is connected to a machine which removes the contents of the uterus by suction. Most women have a light general anaesthetic or a local anaesthetic and are able to go home the same day or the next morning. After 12 weeks the safest method of abortion is called a 'D and C' (Dilation and Curettage), although you can also have this for other reasons. This is normally done under a light general anaesthetic, and involves dilating the cervix and then gently scraping the lining of the uterus with a metal instrument to remove the contents. It's likely that you'll have to stay in hospital overnight.

After 16 weeks abortions can be carried out by using injections of chemicals that make the uterus contract causing the contents to be expelled from the vagina. This is a form of labour induced under sedation or with pain killers, which usually lasts anything from 6 to 24 hours and is more physically and emotionally distressing. At the moment the legal limit for abortion in the UK is 28 weeks (in practice most doctors will not do one after 24 weeks). An operation like a Caesarean section can also be done at a late stage of pregnancy, if other methods are not possible. This is called a hysterotomy and involves making a cut through the abdominal wall and uterus to remove the foetus.

The unsympathetic attitude of some doctors and long waiting lists for beds in hospitals, mean that many women who want abortions have to go as private patients. If you can't pay organisations like the Pregnancy Advisory

Service may be able to provide a loan or, in some cases, arrange for you to have an abortion free on the NHS. If you have a private abortion it's worthwhile asking when you have to pay so you are aware of when it's going to have to be done, as it can be upsetting, or maybe a friend could deal with the money side of things for you. It's a good idea having somebody with you to give you support and to take you home afterwards – so long as their being there doesn't upset you or cause you to worry about how they are feeling.

Don't be surprised if you cry after you wake up from the anaesthetic – this is a very common reaction. Most women have mixed feelings and it is not unusual to feel sad and depressed as well as relieved. These feelings of guilt, sadness and loss are usually short-lived, but if you do continue to feel upset it may help to talk about it with a friend, doctor or counsellor. Afterwards you may feel tired and have some pain and bleeding, but this usually only lasts a day or two. Most women recover from an abortion very quickly, although late abortions take longer. If you continue to bleed, have cramping pains or develop a fever, then see a doctor. It's very easy to get an infection afterwards so if you notice any unusual discharge or other symptoms of vaginal infection, you should have a check-up. To safeguard against this, don't have intercourse or insert anything in your vagina, including tampons, for 6 weeks after the abortion.

There are several illnesses that you can get by having sex with an infected person. Some infections, like thrush, can develop without having sex, but can also be passed on to your partner. If you think you might have a sexually transmitted disease (STD) you should arrange to see a doctor and you should not have sex until you have discovered what is wrong, otherwise you could infect your partner. You could go to your own doctor, but she or he may not be very knowledgeable about STDs and you might be worried about confidentiality. STD clinics give completely free and confidential advice and

●

Having to hand over the money there and then was awful; it made me feel as if I was so callous and cold.

●

I talked to someone I know who's had an abortion. I wanted to have some idea before I went of what might happen.

●

Going to the STD clinic

When is there something wrong?

If you have some of these symptoms then it's likely you have an infection (you should not have sex until you have seen a doctor):

unusual discharge from your vagina (or your partner's penis or vagina)

sores or blisters on your genitals

rashes, itchiness on or around your genitals

the urge to urinate more frequently

discomfort, pain or a burning sensation when you pee

blood in your urine

pain in the lower abdomen

any unusual lump or swelling

pain with penetration

treatment and they are really the best places to go to. (Some clinics give you a number so that other patients won't recognise you by name, or you could give a false name.) The doctors there are used to seeing people with sexually transmitted diseases and are experts in diagnosing what's wrong. You do not need a referral from your GP, you can just ring up and make an appointment or, if you are prepared to wait, some clinics will see you that day. There are STD clinics in most cities and towns – sometimes they're called special clinics, VD clinics or genito-urinary clinics. They are usually attached to the largest hospital in the area; look in the phone book under VD, STD clinic, genito-urinary clinic (GU clinic) or under the local health authority.

Most STDs can be treated easily and quickly but it's important that you go for treatment immediately you notice that anything is wrong. You should also see a doctor if your partner has any symptoms (and they should too!). The longer you leave it the more you put your health at risk as well as, with some infections, your chances of having children.

What puts a lesbian at risk of getting STDs?
It doesn't mean that you are immune from sexually transmitted diseases if you only have sex with women. For instance, if you or your partner's fingers, or an object such as a vibrator, are covered with infected vaginal or cervical secretions and come into contact with the mucous membranes of the genitals or anus there is a risk of transmitting sexually transmitted infections, including herpes, thrush, trichomoniasis and HIV (see later). Oral sex and vagina-to-vagina rubbing might also allow the transmission of herpes, gonorrhoea, vaginal infections and HIV. The following chapter discusses ways of reducing the risk of getting a sexually transmitted infection if you make love with another woman, as well as other issues of relevance to lesbians. Also, like any woman, you will be at risk if you have sex with men and don't take precautions to make it safe.

Many people are reluctant to go to an STD clinic. Even the most assertive woman can find herself feeling embarrassed and uncomfortable at the thought. One reason why people react in this way is the attitudes we have about sex: the old idea that having a sexually transmitted disease is some kind of punishment for being immoral or sinful is still around, as we have seen in the judgemental way AIDS is often talked about. As a result, we can end up feeling guilty and ashamed if we develop an infection or illness that is passed on during sex.

It's a good idea, if you are feeling nervous, to take a friend along with you. But in any case it's important to remember that doctors in STD clinics see hundreds of cases every week. They are used to people feeling embarrassed and are not going to be shocked by what you tell them. It is part of their job to help put you at your ease. Another common worry that people have is that they might bump into someone they know – but how can they say they saw you at the STD clinic unless they say they were there too!

If you know what to expect it can help to feel more at ease. You will be asked to give your name, address and date of birth, together with some brief details of your medical history. It is up to you whether you give your real name but it is important to say if you are allergic to penicillin or any other medicines. You should also tell them if you are taking any medication. You'll be asked why you've come to the clinic and whether you have any symptoms and what they are. They will also ask whether you've made love with anyone you know has an infection, what contraception you use and other questions about your sex-life, such as when you last had sex, what kind of sexual contact you've had (whether you've had cunnilingus or fellatio, vaginal or anal intercourse), and whether you've had any other partners in the last few months. It is important to tell the doctor whether you are pregnant, or if you might be, as this may affect the kind of treatment you are given. All the information you give will be treated as confidential.

●

People assume if you have a sexually transmitted disease that that means you are bad; promiscuous; dirty; it serves you right for getting it.

●

When I first went to a special clinic I was scared not only that I might have some incurable disease, but also in case someone saw me and thought I was 'unclean'.

●

What will they do at the clinic?

●

I chose to go to a clinic instead of my own doctor because there's a certain anonymity about an STD clinic and whatever it is you've got doesn't appear on your medical records.

●

49

●

My doctor asked me questions about how regular my period was, and was I taking any form of contraception? I felt slightly anxious and panicky; I could have said I'm a lesbian or that I don't need to use any form of contraception when I have sex. That would have been much easier. I didn't want to say I was a lesbian in case it went down on my medical records.

●

When I told the doctor I was a lesbian she was OK. She didn't make me feel as if I was doing anything unusual.

●

If your partner is a woman it can be more difficult. Many doctors simply assume that you must be heterosexual but if you know what to expect and are prepared for certain questions it can make the appointment easier to cope with. If say you are a lesbian and you are not at an STD clinic, it might go down on your medical records, but if you state that you are celibate the doctor may not diagnose an STD. If you decide that you do not want to come out, you could say that you don't need to use any form of contraception because you don't have sexual intercourse with men.

After the initial interview, you'll be examined. Many women feel nervous or embarrassed at the thought of a vaginal examination, when someone looks at a part of our body we are not used to showing to anyone but our sexual partners. It helps to remember that the doctor or nurse will have done this many times before. You can take a friend or your partner if you feel uneasy or ask to be examined by a woman when you make an appointment.

The doctor will check for any signs of infection such as rashes or sores on your genitals and will feel for any swelling or inflammation inside by gently inserting a finger into your vagina. You'll also be given a cervical smear test. A speculum is inserted into the vagina to hold the vaginal walls open to allow the cervix to be seen properly and for a small spatula to scrape off a few cells from the cervix (speculums come in different sizes – ask for a smaller one if you feel the need). The whole process only takes a couple of minutes and, although it may be a little uncomfortable, if you can relax it is usually painless. Some women find it easier lying on their side, rather than on their back, so ask about this. Asking the doctor to explain what she or he is doing may also help you to relax because you are more likely to feel tense if you don't feel you have any control over what's happening. Swabs are taken from the vagina and, if you've had anal or oral sex, swabs will be taken from your throat and rectum too. You may also be asked for a urine sample and, whatever your symptoms, you'll be given a blood test for such things as syphilis and hepatitis B.

There are some things you may not be tested for. For instance, you won't necessarily be tested for herpes and if you want to know whether you have been infected with HIV, you'll have to ask for the HIV antibody test. The arguments for and against taking the HIV antibody test are discussed on page 71. If you are worried about AIDS, or if you are not sure about why the doctor is doing something or what tests are being conducted, you should ask.

You may be able to have your results immediately, depending on what tests have been carried out, or you may have to wait a week or two to be told what treatment, if any, is needed. Until you find out whether you do have an infection which can be sexually transmitted you should not have sex that could put your partner at risk.

If you do have a sexually transmitted disease you will be advised to tell those you might have passed it on to. Some clinics, in order to try to prevent the spread of more serious sexually transmitted diseases like AIDS and gonorrhoea, will ask you for the names of the people you have recently had sex with. This is so they can get in touch with them to let them know they may have a sexually transmitted disease, which not only could seriously affect their own health but anyone they have sex with. Even if you have been cured you could become infected again if you have sex with them. But it is your decision whether or not to give the clinic any names; no one can make you tell them.

If you decide not to tell the clinic, it is vital that you tell the people involved. Anyone you might have infected should go to a clinic for treatment too. Don't rely on them finding out for themselves: with many sexually transmitted diseases there are no visible symptoms and a person may have no idea that they have an infection. They may be passing it on to other sexual partners.

•

I felt less vulnerable about having an internal this time because I didn't have to take off all my clothes, and it was a woman doctor.

•

I know I should go see a doctor for a check up, but I'm a bit nervous about having an internal examination.

•

If I could have been involved in pushing the speculum in, perhaps if I had held onto it or held the doctor's hand, I think I would have felt more in control and been able to relax more.

•

If you have an infection

•

When I had a vaginal infection putting anything inside me was really painful, and for a long time after I didn't want to have penetration in case it hurt.

•

Somehow being examined I felt like a piece of meat and that's what it would be like having sex again. It would be like someone examining you.

•

I wasn't in a long-term relationship at the time and I felt that somehow it would be 'promiscuous' to have sex with someone. I felt I should have this period of not doing it.

•

It can come as a shock to learn that you have a sexually transmitted disease. If you've been in a relationship where you've both agreed only to have sex with each other you may feel upset or angry, wondering how you came to be infected. But before you jump to any conclusions and start making accusations, it's important to remember that some infections can occur for other reasons besides having sex (see pages 53–61). Also, you or your partner might have contracted an infection in a previous relationship and not had any symptoms until now.

You may feel guilty and blame yourself. No illness is a punishment; viruses and bacteria cause such diseases rather than 'bad' behaviour, and so having an infection does not mean that you are 'dirty', 'immoral' or 'promiscuous'. Sexually transmitted diseases are a common fact of life and anyone who is sexually active is potentially at risk.

All sorts of other thoughts may go through your mind besides, how have I caught it? How serious is it? Is it possible I've given it to anyone else? Will it affect my health in future? Can it be treated? What effect is this going to have on my relationships? The staff at the STD clinic, or possibly your own doctor, should be able to help answer these and similar sorts of questions. One issue that can be particularly difficult to deal with is sex. Some women do not want to make love with anyone for a long time afterwards, even if they've been treated and they are completely clear, because they feel 'dirty'. Others may be worried about infecting someone else, or they may be worried about being infected again.

Although having HIV or some other infections may mean making changes in your sexual habits, it needn't mean no more sex. You can have sex providing you make love in ways that do not allow the infection to be passed on. Ways of reducing the risk of getting HIV and other sexually transmitted diseases, or of infecting someone else, are discussed in Chapters 3 and 4.

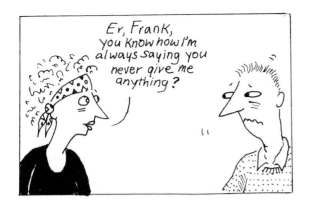

Telling someone you have a sexually transmitted disease is never easy, but it is more or less difficult depending on how serious a disease it is, how you got the infection and, if it was through having sex, who gave it to you. If you are in a relationship and you haven't told your partner you've been sleeping with someone else, you're going to have to discuss more than just a visit to the STD clinic. Alternatively, if you've only had sex with one partner you may feel too upset or angry to be able to tell them you have an infection which, knowingly or not, they have passed on to you. The important thing to get across is that you are telling them for their own health's sake and, so that they don't put anyone else at risk, they should go to the clinic since they might need treatment too.

How to tell someone you have a sexually transmitted disease

WHAT SAFER SEX CAN HELP PROTECT YOU FROM

GONORRHOEA

Usually during vaginal or anal intercourse. You can also become infected by having oral sex with an infected man or – although this seems to happen only very rarely – a woman.

How do you get it?

Most men with gonorrhoea develop a thick, yellowish discharge from the tip of their penis and they experience pain or a burning feeling when they urinate. There are often no symptoms with women. When symptoms do

Symptoms

53

occur, usually 2 to 10 days after being infected, they may include increased vaginal discharge, pain or a burning sensation when peeing, stomach pains and sometimes discharge and itching in the anus (even if you never had anal intercourse). Gonorrhoea passed on during oral sex can cause a sore throat. If it goes untreated it can lead to inflammation of the reproductive organs which may, eventually, cause infertility.

Treatment   Gonorrhoea is easily treated with antibiotics.

SYPHILIS

How do you get it?   It is usually passed on during vaginal or anal intercourse but it can be transmitted from a pregnant woman to her baby. As pregnant women are automatically tested for syphilis this is extremely rare.

Symptoms   Stage 1.   A few weeks after you've been infected, a painless sore usually appears, most often on the genitals but occasionally on the mouth, urethra or anus. The sore usually lasts 2 to 3 weeks.
Stage 2.   Two to 6 months after infection, a rash appears on various parts of the body and you get flu-like symptoms, such as fever, headaches, aching joints, and a sore throat. These symptoms eventually disappear and the disease becomes latent.
Stage 3.   If left untreated syphilis can cause insanity, blindness, paralysis and, eventually, death, but this is very rare.

Treatment   Syphilis is extremely easy to cure with antibiotics and it is very rare for anyone who has it to progress to the later stages. If you go to an STD clinic they will automatically test you for syphilis.

CHLAMYDIA

How do you get it?   During vaginal or anal intercourse and (less often) oral sex with an infected person. A pregnant woman can pass it on to her baby in the

54

form of eye diseases and pneumonia.

Symptoms

Women rarely have any symptoms. When they do these can include a cloudy discharge from the vagina, irritation or soreness in the genital area, frequent need to urinate and pain when you do. In men the symptoms are a discharge from the penis and a burning sensation when peeing.

If it goes untreated chlamydia can lead to more serious complications, such as pelvic inflammatory disease (PID). In severe cases this can make a woman infertile. Women who use an IUD as a form of contraception are more at risk of this happening.

Treatment

As the symptoms are similar to a number of other infections you should ask to be tested for chlamydia to avoid being misdiagnosed. Chlamydia is very easy to cure with antibiotics when it is caught early.

THRUSH (CANDIDA)

How do you get it?

This is a type of yeast infection caused by an organism which usually lives harmlessly in the vagina and rectum. You can get thrush without ever having had sex with someone. If the vagina becomes less acidic by taking antibiotics or during a period, the organism may spread, causing an infection, and there is a greater likelihood of getting thrush if you are pregnant, run down, under stress or experience a change of diet. It is also easily transmitted during sex. Using a condom will reduce the risk of transmission during vaginal or anal intercourse. Similarly, washing your hands after touching your own or your partner's genitals will help prevent thrush being transferred by fingers. Don't share towels or flannels if you have thrush, or if your partner does.

Symptoms

A thick, white yeasty-smelling discharge from your vagina, which can look a bit like cottage cheese. You will probably feel itchy and sore around the opening to the vagina and perhaps around your anus. It may also hurt to pee.

55

Treatment The treatment for thrush usually consists of pessaries that slowly dissolve, or a cream that you insert into your vagina with an applicator. Some home remedies for thrush include putting plain live yogurt into the vagina (you can use a tampon to keep it in place) and adding vinegar to the bath water. Both these methods work by making the vagina more acidic.

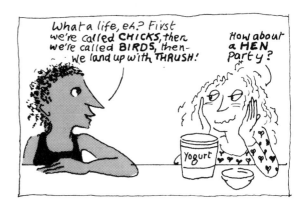

You can also help to prevent thrush by being careful to wipe yourself from front to back after you've been to the toilet, to avoid transmitting thrush from your anus to your vagina, by wearing cotton underwear, avoiding using bubble baths and scented soaps, taking steps to reduce stress, and eating a diet low in sugar and yeast.

GARDNERELLA
(sometimes called non-specific vaginitis)

How do you get it? Gardnerella can be sexually transmitted, but like thrush it can occur spontaneously if the vagina becomes less acidic, such as just before a period.

Symptoms There may be no symptoms at all or you may develop a grey, fishy-smelling discharge. It may also hurt when you pee.

Treatment The usual treatment is a course of antibiotics.

TRICHOMONIASIS

It is caused by a micro-organism which can live harmlessly in the rectum but often causes an infection when it lives in the vagina. It is usually sexually transmitted during intercourse.

How do you get it?

You usually have a thin, foamy, yellowish-green or greyish vaginal discharge that smells rather fishy and is very often itchy. The vulva may be sore and inflamed, and it may hurt to pee. Women who have trichomoniasis often also have gonorrhoea.

Symptoms

If you have trichomoniasis you will usually be prescribed a drug called Metronidazole, which is taken orally.

Treatment

CERVICAL CANCER

Cervical cancer is a cancer which starts in the cervix or neck of the womb (uterus). Nobody yet fully understands what causes it but there is some evidence to suggest that it may be linked to a virus which can be passed on during vaginal intercourse. A number of risk factors have been identified. These include: having vaginal intercourse in your early teens, especially if you didn't use a condom or a cap; having unprotected intercourse with several partners (or if a partner has); being a smoker; becoming pregnant in your teens; having sexually transmitted diseases, especially genital warts and herpes; several pregnancies; having vaginal intercourse with a man who has a history of sexually transmitted diseases.

If you fall into any or all of these categories it does not mean that you are going to develop cervical cancer, but it does mean that your chances are higher. Because of the increased risk you should have a cervical smear test *every year*, just to be on the safe side.

You can't tell by just looking at your cervix whether you've got cancer but it can be picked up by a simple test called a cervical smear. (What happens when you have a cervical smear test is described in more detail on page 50.) This

How do you know if you've got it?

only takes a couple of minutes and should not hurt. The cells from your cervix are examined to see whether they are normal or if they are showing changes that could develop into cancer.

How often should I have a smear test?
You should have a smear test soon after you first have vaginal intercourse and then, if the smear is normal, every 3 years. Women who have never had sexual intercourse should still have regular smear tests, especially if they are over 35. You should be tested at least once a year if you have previously had a positive smear result, if you experience unexplained vaginal bleeding outside your period, if you have an unusual discharge, if you have genital warts or herpes, or if you are at increased risk for getting this cancer for some other reason.

Where can I get the test?
Unfortunately, GPs only get paid for doing a cervical smear test if you are over 35 (or if you have 3 or more children) and are tested every 5 years. This is based on the fact that most women who get cancer of the cervix are over 35 and that it takes from 3 to 5 years and sometimes longer for the cancer cells to grow. Recently, however, there has been a rapid increase in a new kind of cervical cancer in young women which appears to progress much faster. For this reason, most doctors will agree to take smears from younger women, as well as doing tests more regularly than every 5 years. Alternatively, you could go to a family planning clinic, STD clinic, or well-woman clinic.

Wherever you go to have a cervical smear taken, you should make sure you find out the result of the test. Sometimes it can take several weeks before the result comes through. If you don't hear anything, don't simply assume everything must be OK, telephone the doctor or clinic to check.

I've never had a smear test. As a lesbian who only has sex with other women, do I need to?
Yes, especially if you are over 35. Although

cervical cancer seems to be linked with vaginal intercourse without a condom, we don't yet fully understand what causes it. Only having had sex with women, or being celibate, may reduce the risks of your developing cervical cancer but it does not mean you don't need to bother to have a smear test. In any case, some lesbians who now only have sex with women used to have sex with men. If this applies to you, especially if you started having unprotected intercourse at a young age, then you may be at increased risk of developing cancer of the cervix.

What happens if the smear is positive?

A negative test result means that the cells look normal and no abnormalities have been found. A positive result means that some abnormal cells have shown up on the test. This does not mean you have cancer. Sometimes the cells return to normal and no treatment is required. If this doesn't happen, the abnormal cells can be destroyed or removed, often without damage to the cervix. This is a quick and simple operation and can usually be done as an out-patient under local anaesthetic. The vast majority of women will be completely cured after their treatment. They will, however, need to have regular smears, at least once a year.

Prevention

You can help prevent cervical cancer by having regular smears. Safer sex also has a major role to play in the prevention of cervical cancer: either by making love in ways that don't involve penetration, or by using a condom or a cap. If you smoke you might also think about trying to stop as this is one of the risk factors.

HERPES

What is it?

This is a very common infection caused by two types of virus. Herpes Type 1 is the virus which causes cold sores, while Herpes Type 2 causes sores on the genitals. Once you have been infected with the virus there is no way of getting rid of it – you are infected for life.

How do you get it?

If you kiss someone who has a cold sore you can

59

become infected with the herpes virus and may develop cold sores yourself. It is also possible to pass on the herpes virus from sores on the mouth to the genital area during oral sex or, more rarely, by transferring the virus from a cold sore onto the genital area by fingers. (You can also give yourself herpes by touching a cold sore on your face and then touching your genitals.) The virus can also be transmitted by having vaginal or anal intercourse with someone who has a herpes sore on the genitals. There is also a risk of infection if you have a cut or sore anywhere on your body which, if you rubbed up against or touched someone's infected genitals, would allow the virus entry into your bloodstream.

A person is normally infectious from just before the blisters appear – an itching or tingling sensation in the genital region is often a warning sign – until the sores are completely healed. However it seems that some people are able to pass on the virus in semen or vaginal/cervical secretions, even when no blisters or sores can be seen.

Women with herpes can pass it on to their newborn babies during the birth. To avoid the possibility of the baby coming into contact with the herpes virus in the vagina, pregnant women who have had herpes at the time of birth are usually advised to have a Caesarean section.

How do you know you've got it?

A few days after having sex with the person who infected you, small painful blisters usually appear on the vaginal lips or anal area. You may experience stinging, tingling or itching. Blisters may also appear on the cervix where they are not painful and you may not know you have them, although you will still be infectious. (In men the blisters most commonly occur on the penis but they can also appear in the urethra or rectum.) Some people develop flu-like symptoms as well. Soon after they appear the blisters burst forming open sores or ulcers and at this stage it may hurt to pee. During this time the virus is most likely to be transmitted sexually. It usually takes 2 or 3 weeks for the herpes sores to disappear. The virus remains in the body and although some people never get herpes again, others have further attacks. These may be triggered by stress, illness, sunburn, exhaustion or having a period. Fortunately, these are usually a lot less painful than the first outbreak and often they get less and less frequent over time.

There is currently no vaccine and no known cure for herpes. A few drugs seem to relieve many of the symptoms and reduce the chances of another attack. Otherwise, self-help measures such as keeping the sores clean and dry, wearing loose clothing and cotton underwear, and using cold, wet compresses to relieve the pain, may help to alleviate the symptoms.

What to do about it if you have it

In women there seems to be an association between herpes and cervical cancer. For this reason, it is advisable for all women who have had genital herpes to have a cervical smear test every year.

You can reduce the risk of getting herpes if you practise safer sex and stick to these guidelines: do not practise oral sex if either of you has a cold sore or a sore on the genital area; do not touch a cold sore or a genital herpes sore and then touch your partner's or your own genitals; do not use spit as a lubricant if either of you has a cold sore. Always wash your hands with soap after touching sores, and don't share towels or flannels. (It's unlikely the virus will be passed on in this way, but it is possible.) Using a condom in conjunction with a spermicide or lubricant that contains nonoxynol-9 can help prevent transmission of herpes during intercourse, but it is not 100% safe. (Nonoxynol-9 has been shown to be effective against the herpes virus.) A man who has herpes may still infect a woman if he has sores at the base of his penis, the part which isn't covered by the condom. And remember that it's also possible that the condom may come off or tear.

Prevention

AIDS

Few people had heard of AIDS before 1981, now almost everyone knows about this new and fatal disease – Acquired Immune Deficiency Syndrome. Most researchers believe that AIDS is caused by a virus called human immunodeficiency virus, or HIV, which damages the body's immune system by attacking a particular group of cells in the bloodstream. When your immune system is working properly it protects you from getting ill: a person with AIDS is vulnerable to a whole range of infections and cancers which the immune system would normally ward off. These illnesses are called 'opportunistic infections', which means that in healthy people they are harmless, but in people whose immune systems are not working properly they cause illness and eventually death. One of the most common of these infections is an unusual form of pneumonia known as pneumocystic carinii pneumonia.

Even if HIV does not affect a person's immune system, it may have other serious consequences. The virus can cause damage to the brain and the central nervous system, which leads to loss of memory, personality changes and dementia. Unlike most other viruses, HIV changes the structure of the cells it attacks. It does this by incorporating its own genetic code into the genetic material of the cells it infects. Viruses which function in this way are called retroviruses. What makes them harder to deal with than other viruses is that the virus becomes part of the cells it infects, and there is no way of getting rid of it. A person who has the HIV virus will probably be infected – and be infectious – for life.

If I'm infected with HIV will I get AIDS?

Many people are confused about the difference between being infected with HIV and having AIDS. People with HIV may have no signs of illness. They may look and feel perfectly healthy, even though they are capable of infecting others with the virus. Others who are infected may develop symptoms that are less serious than AIDS itself such as swollen lymph glands, diarrhoea, thrush in their mouth, weight loss and fatigue. How many of those who have the HIV virus will eventually go on to develop AIDS is still uncertain. It seems that about 15 to 30% of people with HIV infection go on to develop AIDS within 5 years of becoming infected and some researchers believe that over a longer period of time as many as 90% may eventually develop the disease, but they still do not know.

As a heterosexual woman how much attention should I pay to AIDS, given that nearly all those who have so far developed AIDS are gay men?
It is true that of the 2,649 cases of AIDS reported in the UK by September 1989, 81% were gay or bisexual men. This is because, for reasons we do not fully understand, gay men were among the first in the USA, Australia and the UK to be infected with the virus. (In other countries, in Central Africa for instance, AIDS seems to primarily affect *heterosexual* women and men.) In recent years however, the rate of increase in AIDS cases among gay men appears to have levelled off, while heterosexual contact with an infected partner has become an increasingly important means of transmission, especially for women. In the USA the percentage of women with AIDS who contracted the virus through sex with an infected man has risen sharply, from 18% of all female cases in 1986, to 29% in 1988. In the UK 45 of the 104 cases of AIDS in women so far reported (43%) have been attributed to heterosexual contact. Of the total number of women known to be antibody positive, 363 (30%) were infected through having unsafe sex with an infected man (September 1989).

A few months ago I made love with a man who I have since found out has the HIV virus. We only had vaginal intercourse once but we didn't use a condom. What are the chances that I could have become infected?
There are estimates which reflect the different

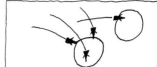
HOW THE VIRUS ATTACKS THE BODY

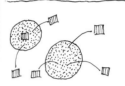

1. Once in the bloodstream HIV attacks a particular group of white cells, called T-helper cells, in the body's defense system

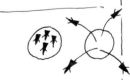

2. T-helper cells alert other white cells to send out antibodies which for some unknown reason do not kill the virus.

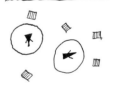

3. The T-helper cells are invaded by HIV which incorporates itself into genetic material of the T-cells.

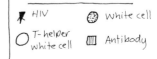

4. HIV can remain dormant for several years before instructing the T-cells to make more viruses, which are then released.

✗ HIV	● white cell
○ T-helper white cell	▥ Antibody

risks but it is vital to remember that, like pregnancy, you only need have intercourse once to become infected. Anyone who has unsafe sex with an infected partner has a small but definite chance, each time, of getting the virus. The more chances you take the greater the likelihood of becoming infected.

Can HIV be passed on through kissing?

No one has ever been known to become infected through kissing and most experts now believe that it is safe to kiss. Although HIV has been found in saliva (spit) it is present in such small amounts that you'd probably need buckets of it to transmit the virus. The only time there may be a risk is if you had sores or cuts in and around your mouth and the saliva contained blood, because infected blood or body fluids have to get into the bloodstream.

Who gets AIDS? In the UK and the USA AIDS has so far mainly affected gay and bisexual men and injecting drug-users. It would be wrong, however, to think that AIDS is not going to happen to you simply because you're not gay and you don't inject drugs. The idea that there are certain 'risk-groups' is dangerously misleading. People get AIDS because of what they do, not because of who they are. We should talk about certain kinds of *behaviour* being 'high risk', rather than certain groups of people. Any woman or man can become infected with HIV and, possibly, develop AIDS, if they behave in ways that allow the virus to get into their body. For example, HIV can be transmitted during anal intercourse. It doesn't matter whether it is a woman and a man or two men doing this (or whether they are gay, bisexual or straight), if one person is infected they could pass on the virus to the other.

Who are the women who get AIDS? Most women diagnosed with AIDS are young, aged between 20 and 35. So far, the number of women with AIDS in Australia and in the UK is low: by September 1989, 104 women were reported as having AIDS and 1,201 had tested positive (the HIV antibody test) in the UK. This makes it difficult to predict what the future pattern of infection among women will be, although the experience of the United States offers some indications. There the number of women with AIDS has increased more than 5 fold in the last 3 years. Of the 109,167 people reported to have AIDS in the United States by September 1989, 9% were women. Half of these were women injecting drug-users; of the rest, 30% contracted the virus through unsafe sex with a man, 11% received transfusions with infected blood. The remaining 7% are women for whom the source of infection has not been identified.

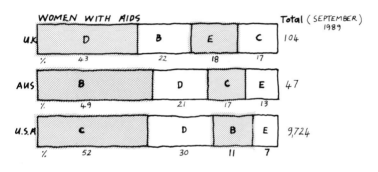

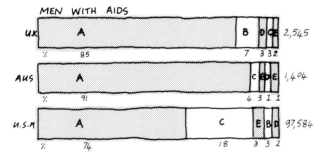

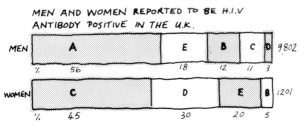

KEY

A Homosexual / bisexual
B Recipients of
   blood products
C I.V. drug users
D Heterosexual
E Miscellaneous

AUS Australia
% Percentage of total

Are lesbians at risk of getting AIDS?

Anyone can become infected with HIV and, possibly, develop AIDS, if they do things that put them at risk of infection. Just because a woman is a lesbian doesn't mean she won't become infected if she has unsafe sex with a man who has the virus, or if she shares equipment to inject drugs. The risk comes from what you do, not how you label yourself.

Is it possible for a woman to sexually transmit HIV to another woman? So far there have been only 2 cases reported where it's thought that the virus may have been passed on sexually from woman to woman. There are 2 reasons why woman to woman transmission is so rare. Firstly, although if you have sex with another woman your lovemaking may include 'penetrative sex', such as a shared vibrator inserted in the vagina or anus, which could transmit the virus, you are not going to be engaging in vaginal or anal intercourse – the main way people become infected with HIV. Secondly, the fact that, at present, a far greater proportion of men are infected than women means that if you have sex with a woman you are less likely to encounter an infected partner than if you have sex with a man.

How is HIV transmitted?

HIV is very fragile and is easily killed outside the body. This is why the virus cannot be passed from one person to another by casual contact such as shaking hands or sharing a meal. If the virus could be contracted through normal daily contact there would be many AIDS cases among health workers or family and friends caring for people with AIDS and this is not so.

Most people contract HIV through having intercourse, vaginal or anal, with someone who is already infected with the virus. For transmission to occur, semen, blood or vaginal and cervical secretions must pass from one person to another, through the moist skin lining in the vagina, rectum or urethra, or via cuts or breaks in the skin or mouth. During intercourse the virus may get into a woman's bloodstream through small cuts or tears in the walls of the vagina or anus, and such small tears, which you are unlikely to notice, happen quite often during intercourse. The virus may also enter the blood through ulcerations of the cervix or by being absorbed through the vaginal walls, which become swollen with blood during sexual arousal. Cuts or open sores on a woman's genital area may also allow semen (or blood) containing the virus to enter the bloodstream. For this reason other untreated sexually transmitted diseases may increase your risk of HIV infection. A woman who has herpes or gonorrhoea, for example, may have genital sores or ulcers which could make it easier for the virus to enter her bloodstream.

Just as a man can transmit the HIV virus to a woman during intercourse, it is also possible for a woman to pass it on to a man. Again, the chances of the virus being transmitted are likely to be far greater if there are cuts or abrasions on a man's penis, or if he has a dry or inflamed urethra which could allow the virus entry into his bloodstream. Because HIV is found in menstrual blood (as it is in all blood) as well as cervical and vaginal secretions, the risk of infection is likely to be greater during a woman's period.

Some researchers believe that the virus is more easily transmitted from a man to a woman than from a woman to a man; this seems logical but it is not conclusive. Whether it is true or not, the fact that, at present, a lot more men than women are infected puts women at greater risk. A woman is more likely to encounter an infected man than a man is an infected woman and this probably explains the larger numbers of hetereosexually-acquired AIDS cases among women. Of the 5,048 reported cases of AIDS in the USA due to heterosexual contact with an infected person, over 59% are women (September, 1989).

Although vaginal or anal intercourse is the main way HIV is passed on from one person to another, it's also possible that other ways of having sex could transmit the virus. Oral sex, for example, is known to transmit most other sexually transmitted diseases, but whether the HIV virus can be transmitted orally is not

You can't contract HIV from:
Toilet seats
Towels
Swimming pools
Telephones
Crockery and cutlery
Shaking hands
Books
Mosquitoes, fleas or other blood-sucking insects
Hugging
Coughs and sneezes

How serious is AIDS?

Since the first cases of AIDS were officially reported in the USA, in 1981, the disease has spread very rapidly. As of September 1989, 142 countries around the world have reported over 182,000 cases of AIDS, although the true figure is probably almost twice that.

The number of new cases of AIDS continues to grow. In the USA, where over 109,000 people have been officially diagnosed as having AIDS, the number of AIDS cases doubles approximately every 12 months. In the UK where there are 2,649 recorded cases, the total number of AIDS cases doubles every 10 months (September, 1989).

In addition to those who have AIDS, between 5 and 10 million people worldwide are infected with HIV. In the UK there are an estimated 50,000 people with HIV.

AIDS is the most serious sexually transmitted disease that we currently face, but it is also possible to prevent. Although there is currently no vaccine against HIV, we can avoid the risk of infection with the virus which causes AIDS by practising safer sex, and by safer drug use.

absolutely clear (see page 99). It seems unlikely, although there may be some risk of infection if there are cuts or sores on a person's mouth, lips, gums or tongue which would allow infected semen, blood or vaginal and cervical fluids to enter the bloodstream. Aside from sexual transmission, the other main way of becoming infected with HIV is if you share needles or any other equipment for mixing and injecting drugs. Once infected this way, anyone can then pass on the virus to their sexual partners if they practise unsafe sex.

In the past some people developed AIDS as a result of being given blood or blood products which had been infected with HIV. Many haemophiliacs, who require treatment with blood products to help their blood to clot, contracted the virus this way. Nowadays all blood donors are screened for HIV and blood products are heat-treated to kill the virus, making them safe to use.

Finally, women who are infected with HIV can pass the virus on to the foetus during pregnancy, via the placenta, or possibly during birth. It is estimated that there is about a 1 in 4 chance of this happening. Because, in a pregnant woman, the immune system is suppressed to stop the body rejecting the foetus, some doctors have suggested that pregnancy might increase the chances of a woman who has the virus going on to develop AIDS. But it now seems that this is probably not the case. The medical advice to women known to be antibody positive is not to have children or, if they are already pregnant, to think about having an abortion. If you are HIV antibody positive you have the right to choose whether or not you have children. Some women do decide to have an abortion; others continue with the pregnancy. Whatever decision a woman makes about having children, it's important that it is her own decision – don't let pressure from your doctor influence you. If you do decide to have a child, discuss how having an infected baby would affect your life and relationships. The virus has been found in breastmilk and women with HIV infection will be advised not to breastfeed their babies until more is known about the possibility of transmission.

Any woman thinking about having a baby by artificial insemination should be aware that the virus has been passed on in this way, and so they should check that the donor they are using has not been infected with HIV. Sperm donors are now tested by clinics offering artificial insemination.

When someone becomes infected with the HIV virus their body reacts by producing antibodies which can be detected in the blood by using the HIV antibody test. This is *not* an 'AIDS test'. The HIV antibody test is a simple blood test which shows whether or not you have the antibodies to the HIV virus. It does not tell you whether you have AIDS or if you will develop AIDS in the future.

How can I tell if I'm infected?

If a test produces a *positive* result it means that you have been infected with the virus at some time, and that antibodies to the virus are in your blood. People who test positive are said to be antibody positive or sero-positive. They could transmit the virus to others if they don't practise safer sex, or if they share needles or other equipment for mixing and injecting drugs. A woman who is antibody positive and becomes pregnant could pass the virus on to her baby.

A negative result means either that you are not infected with HIV, or that your body has not made antibodies yet. It takes, on average, 2 to 3 months from infection for antibodies to HIV to develop. For this reason you might want to wait 3 months before having the test but during this period you should not do anything that would put you at risk of HIV or of infecting someone else.

If you do test negative it doesn't mean that you are immune to AIDS *or that you won't become infected with HIV in future.* To avoid future infection you should practise safer sex if you think your partner might be infected, or if you are not sure, and, if you inject drugs, stop sharing your 'works'.

I had an affair some time ago with a bisexual man and am worried about AIDS. What should I do?

If you are worried about past sexual relationships you should carry out a 'risk assessment'. The likelihood of your being infected will depend on a number of factors. When and where did the relationship take place? Your chances of meeting an infected man in London in 1989 were much higher than, for instance, they were in 1980. Was it someone whose activities put them at risk of infection? Just because someone is bisexual doesn't mean they are automatically at risk but if your partner was having anal intercourse regularly with other men and being penetrated, without using a condom, then he could have become infected with the virus. Was he ever a drug-user? If he was, he could have become infected by sharing equipment.

What kinds of sex did you have? If you had vaginal or anal intercourse, did you use a condom? How often did you have unsafe sex with one another? Did you, at that time, have a vaginal infection or untreated sexually transmitted disease which might have made it easier for the virus to get into the bloodstream?

If you feel that you might be infected you should practise safer sex to avoid the possibility of passing the virus on to someone else. The same precautions will protect you from becoming infected in future if you don't have the virus. You might also consider taking the HIV antibody test.

Should I take the test?

If you are thinking of taking the test you should start by asking yourself a number of questions. Why do you want the test? What do you expect to gain by being tested? What happens if the result turns out to be positive? How will knowing you are positive or negative affect your life? Do you need to know the result to help you change your behaviour? *Whatever you decide you should practise safer sex.*

Where can I take the test?

You can take the test, which is free, at your local STD clinic or, alternatively, your doctor can

THE HIV ANTIBODY TEST

What are the disadvantages of having the HIV antibody test?

Many people assume knowing their test result has to be better than not knowing, but this is not always the case.

If you test positive you may become extremely anxious, worrying about whether you will become ill and eventually die of AIDS.

If you are tested by your GP it may go down on your medical records and you may find it difficult to get life insurance and mortgages (the STD clinic will test in confidence).

You may be discriminated against if it is known that you have the virus; in some cases people have been evicted from their homes or have lost their jobs. Others have been rejected by their families and friends.

If you test negative you may assume you are no longer at risk and that you don't need to practise safer sex. Whatever the result the advice is the same: Practise safer sex.

What are the advantages of having the HIV antibody test?

If you think you might have been at risk of infection, it *may* put your mind at ease.

You may find it easier to practise safer sex (or safer drug-use) if you know that you are infected with HIV. *But you should be doing this anyway!*

If you do have the virus you may be able to alter your lifestyle in ways that may reduce your risk of becoming ill, as well as infecting someone else.

If you do develop symptoms you are likely to be diagnosed quicker and start treatment earlier.

You may want to be tested if you are pregnant and you think you are at risk, or you are considering having a baby (see page 68). If you are going to have the test in order to decide whether or not to go ahead with having a child, make sure your partner is tested as well or, if you are using artificial insemination, make sure that the donor has been screened for HIV infection.

Many of the drugs that are currently being tested are aimed at stopping the HIV virus from reproducing itself once it has entered the body. In future those who know they are positive may be able to benefit from such treatment, which could prolong their good health.

Whether you decide to take the test or not, you should practise safer sex to make sure you don't give or get the virus.

arrange the test. It can take 2 or 3 weeks to get the result.

The advantage of going to a clinic is that testing can be done in strictest confidence. If you go to your doctor for the HIV antibody test the result may be entered in your medical records, which employers and insurance companies could have access to in future. Another reason for being tested at a clinic which specialises in diseases like AIDS, is that you will probably be more likely to get the counselling you need to help you decide whether or not to take the test. It is essential that you discuss your reasons for wanting the test, and the arguments for and against it, before being tested. For more information contact one of the AIDS organisations listed on page 161.

If you have some of the symptoms listed it does not necessarily mean that you have AIDS. Many of these symptoms are also symptoms of other illnesses. For instance, fever and weight loss are much more likely to be symptoms of stress, exhaustion or of a cold coming on, and swollen glands may mean that you've got glandular fever. If you do have some of these symptoms and are worried that you may have been infected with HIV you should see a doctor, preferably at an STD clinic. Some people feel nervous or uncomfortable about attending an STD clinic, in which case it helps to know what to expect when you go (see page 49). You can find the address of your nearest clinic by looking in the phone book under STD (sexually transmitted diseases), VD (venereal disease), genito-urinary clinic, or local health authority. You could also contact one of the AIDS organisations listed on page 161 for information and advice.

Can AIDS be treated?

There is no known cure for AIDS. Certain drugs, such as AZT (Azidothymidine), may help to slow down the progress of the disease, but there is currently no treatment that will restore the immune system or destroy the HIV virus once it is in a person's body. Despite this, people with AIDS are often successfully treated for many of the infections and cancers associated with AIDS, and they lead active lives for long periods of time. But they still have AIDS and will be susceptible to further infections and cancers which will probably eventually cause their death. Most people diagnosed with AIDS die within 5 years.

Is there a vaccine?
At present there is no vaccine to stop AIDS developing. Although work on this is progressing, researchers face many difficulties and it's unlikely that a vaccine will be developed for some years. Even if one is produced tomorrow it will take years to test whether it is safe to use.

I've just started going out with a man who I like and want to have sex with. My friend says I should insist on him using a condom. Is this a good idea?
Yes. You don't know whether he has a sexually transmitted infection, like HIV, and you certainly can't tell from what he looks like. Just because you've decided to go out with him doesn't mean that he'd automatically tell you if he has – and he might not even know. Using a condom will reduce your risk of becoming infected with HIV or other sexually transmitted infections. It may also protect you from cervical cancer and, if used properly in combination

What are the symptoms of AIDS?
The general symptoms of AIDS may include:

Sudden loss of a lot of weight

Swollen glands, especially in the groin, neck or armpits

Persistent diarrhoea

Shortness of breath, together with a dry irritating cough that won't go away

Profound fatigue, which lasts for weeks, with no obvious cause

Fever, shaking chills or drenching night sweats

Dark pink or purple spots, like small bruises, that do not go away. This is a rare form of skin cancer called Kaposi's sarcoma. For reasons that are not fully understood, very few women with AIDS get this.

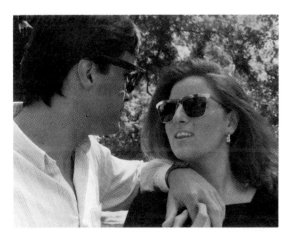

'Let's make it safe'

with a spermicide, it is a very effective method of contraception, without any risk to your health. You might also want to discuss safe ways of making love without having intercourse. After all, safer sex isn't just about using a condom!

Talking about safer sex can imply that you don't trust someone, but really it means that you care enough to be concerned about each other's health and pleasure. If he refuses to discuss safer sex, or puts you down for suggesting it, what does that say about his attitude towards you and your feelings? Do you want to begin a relationship with someone who doesn't care about you enough to make love in ways you *both* want and enjoy?

Prevention Though there is no vaccine and no known cure for AIDS, it is a preventable disease. We know how the virus is transmitted. We don't need to be frightened of AIDS or think that it means no more sex. All we have to do is apply what is known about AIDS to our lives, by practising safer sex or by changing our drug habits. The problem for most of us is that even though we may understand the need for safer sex, we find it difficult to change our sexual habits and talk to our partners about it. The following chapter looks at ways in which you can have a safe and enjoyable sex life.

CHAPTER THREE

SAFER
SEX

What does the phrase safer sex mean to you?
Do you see it as sticking to one partner, using
condoms, giving up sex altogether or as a fun
way of expressing your sexuality? It could mean
any of these and many other things, but
whatever images and feelings it conjures up for
you, it's important to know which are good
strategies for preventing sexually transmitted
infections or unplanned pregnancy, and which
are risky.

What is safer sex?

There is nothing wrong or abnormal about not
wanting to have sexual relationships, and that
includes not wanting to masturbate. We
shouldn't feel forced to have sex, and it is
possible to choose celibacy without feeling that
you are a failure at relationships or are no
longer attractive and desirable. Celibacy can be
a time for learning about yourself and what you
need from relationships, of discovering a sense
of independence and individuality, of freeing
time and energy for friendships and new pur-
suits. For some people, however, it is not a
positive choice; it is a decision based on fear –
often a fear of AIDS.

Celibacy

   Certainly celibacy is a way of protecting
yourself from AIDS and other sexually
transmitted diseases (although you would still
be at risk of HIV infection if you shared equip-

ment to inject drugs). And, if you have previously had sex with men, you no longer have to worry about pregnancy or the health risks associated with various forms of contraception. Celibacy can also be a way of protecting yourself emotionally, as well as physically, and this might be important if, for example, you have been abused in a relationship.

If you are going to abstain from sex out of fear of AIDS remember that it is not necessarily going to make your desire for relationships suddenly disappear. There is a danger that you may end up in situations where you find yourself throwing caution to the wind and taking risks. Celibacy can be a choice, but it is one that is unrealistic for most people. It is also unnecessary; you don't *have* to give up all forms of sex to prevent transmission of HIV, or other sexual risks. There are many ways of making love safely – as you'll see from this chapter.

Being monogamous

For some people monogamy means having one sexual partner for life, for others it means being faithful to your partner for however long the relationship lasts. On this basis, you could have a series of relationships, one after the other, and still regard yourself as monogamous. But because of the long incubation period of the progression from HIV infection to AIDS, this pattern of 'serial monogamy' might put you at risk. Staying with one sexual partner will not prevent transmission of HIV, or sexually transmitted diseases, if you or your partner are infected and you make love in ways that allow transmission of the virus.

If you are in a relationship where *neither* of you have had sex with anyone else since the late 1970s, and neither of you have shared equipment to inject drugs, received a blood transfusion or are a haemophiliac, then it is extremely unlikely that you are infected. But if either of you has had unsafe sex with another person in that time, or put yourself at risk in other ways, it is possible that you could be infected – which is why it is dangerous to believe that if you are monogamous then you are safe. Your partner may have done something, perhaps before he or she met you, and seen no reason to tell you. You could both take the HIV antibody test at the beginning of a relationship but whatever the result, you still need to trust one another to be totally honest about other sexual relationships or injecting drugs – something that is not always easy to do, however much we might want to.

Lifelong monogamy is not a realistic risk reduction strategy for many people. Sexual relationships end for all sorts of reasons and people develop new ones, and of course we do not always find Mr or Ms Right the first or second time and sometimes we don't even want to! For some of us, being monogamous is not an option because we don't want to limit ourselves to having sex with only one person.

Some people believe that it is only people who are 'promiscuous' who get AIDS or other sexually transmitted diseases. (Although the meaning of 'promiscuous' seems to vary – it usually refers to someone who has sex more than we do!) It's true that the more sexual partners you have the greater your chances are of encountering someone with the HIV virus or a sexually transmitted disease, it is also possible to have sex safely with different partners, but whether or not you are at greater risk of infection will depend on what you do together. Similarly, reducing the number of sexual partners you have will not significantly reduce your risk of infection if you don't practise safer sex; it only takes one infected partner.

Fewer sexual partners

One strategy that was recommended early on in the AIDS epidemic was not to have sex with people from so called 'high-risk' groups and this included gay or bisexual men, injecting drug-users, haemophiliacs and prostitutes. Nowadays the idea of high-risk groups is recognised as being very misleading. It may allow some people to think that they won't become infected with HIV simply because they are not gay or an injecting drug-user, or that their partners aren't.

While it's true to say that some people are

Choose your partner carefully

77

more at risk of HIV infection than others, it's not because they belong to a certain social group. Some women inject drugs and share needles but don't consider themselves to be drug-*users*; a lot of men have unprotected penetrative sex with other men but don't see themselves as gay or even bisexual. They may not think they are at risk but they are! Equally, you shouldn't automatically assume that people who fall into the so-called high-risk categories will be doing things which put them at risk. Many gay men, for instance, practise safer sex; not all injecting drug-users share needles.

The only way to be certain of reducing your risk, with any partner, is to practise safer sex.

Know your partner well

The strategy of asking your partner about their sexual history won't stop you from becoming infected with HIV or anything else. Although it is a very good idea in practice it means you have to trust your partner to be honest with you. Some people are reluctant to discuss their past sex-lives (or drug experiences). They may be ashamed, embarrassed, or feel that if they told the truth they would damage the relationship or ruin their chances of sex. If someone thinks that the only way to persuade you to have sex with them is to lie, or to be economical with the truth, you could be at risk.

It's safer if you use a condom

Safer sex isn't just about using a condom but if your lovemaking does include having penetrative sex, condoms can make it safer. Vaginal intercourse with a condom is not completely safe, as people sometimes do not use them properly and they can come off during intercourse or they can split. But condoms can reduce the risk of transmitting HIV and most sexually transmitted diseases, as well as offering some protection against cervical cancer and pregnancy. It's important to realise that most condoms are designed for vaginal intercourse and may therefore offer less protection when used for anal penetration. (Condoms break more often in anal sex because your anus doesn't lubricate itself.) For a full discussion of the part condoms can play in safer sex see pages 112–27.

Despite the cautions about taking the test (see page 71), this is a safer sex option which may appeal to some people. In some parts of the world it is one that is encouraged through the establishment of HIV antibody negative dating clubs. But, of course, it is not a strategy for reducing risk that can be totally relied upon. Just because you and your partner are antibody negative now doesn't mean that you won't be at risk of HIV infection in future if either of you have unsafe sex with someone who may be infected, or if either of you share equipment to inject drugs.

I only have sex with people who are antibody negative

These are examples of strategies for reducing risk but most of them are either not very good or they are unrealistic for many people. How else can we make the sexual relationships we enjoy safer and still have fun?

Safer sex

More important than who you have sex with, or how often, is the way you make love. For example, unprotected vaginal intercourse puts you at risk of unplanned pregnancies and unprotected vaginal or anal intercourse puts you at risk of sexually transmitted diseases. And while there are many ways in which sexual abuse can occur, when women are coerced or forced into having sex they do not want, it often involves penetration.

You could decide to stop intercourse completely and there are lots of exciting ways to enjoy sex. Stroking, caressing, mutual masturbation and other safe ways of making love don't always get the press they deserve because when people think of sex they think of intercourse. But it would be wrong to assume that this is what women always like or want sexually. Lots of women get as much pleasure, or more, from sex that does not involve penetration. There is nothing unusual or abnormal about this and we shouldn't assume that some men don't prefer rubbing, stroking and caressing to intercourse as well. Intercourse is only one way of enjoying sex – you have your hands,

79

your fingers, your mouth and the rest of your body to make love with.

Safer sex is not only a way of caring for our health and psychological well-being, it's an opportunity to explore new ways of making love too. It is easy to get into a sexual rut – to make love in the same way, in the same positions, doing the same things, whispering the same sweet nothings, at the same times of the day or night and in familiar settings. Safer sex is a chance to bring new thrills and excitement to our love-lives, to do what feels good rather than what's expected of us! It's an opportunity to increase the enjoyment we get from sex by becoming more aware of the sensual and erotic potential of the whole body, rather than just concentrating on the genitals. It can also be

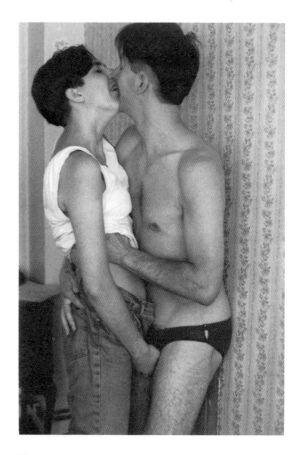

about showing your partner what you do and what you don't like.

For some of us safer sex is already a part of our way of life. For others who are just beginning to think about it, this chapter is about helping you decide what this is going to mean in *practice*. Like anything else, sex is what you make it. This is not an exhaustive list – use your imagination! The possibilities for safer sex are practically endless.

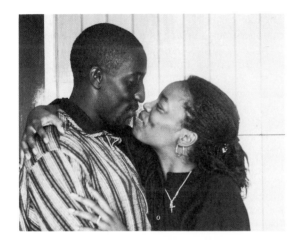

Sex can be a lot of fun, but it also involves risks. Not everyone will want or be able to give up intercourse or to make the same changes to their sex-lives. Much depends on the kind of sexual relationships you have, how much control you have within them and what you and your partner enjoy doing. Similarly, it's not possible to generalize about safer sex in every situation. The risk associated with a certain kind of behaviour may change depending on the circumstances, for example, oral sex with a woman is more risky, in terms of HIV transmission, if she is having her period (see page 99). If you have an eczema-like rash on your hands it will increase the risk of transmission of HIV during vaginal or anal penetration with fingers.

The emotional risk involved in sex will also vary. Sharing sexual fantasies, for instance,

Do it safely!

may be extremely arousing and feel very safe – but if those fantasies involve violence, sharing them may be disturbing. Ultimately, it will be you and your sexual partner who will decide what is an acceptable amount of risk (see page 103).

Mutual masturbation

Using your hands to enjoy touching and stroking each other's genitals is for many people one of the easiest ways of having an orgasm. This is called 'mutal masturbation', but the trouble with this phrase is that it suggests that what you are doing together is an imitation of masturbation, which it's not. What does the term mutual masturbation include?

You could take turns at touching each other, you could touch each other at the same time or find it arousing to stimulate your partner while touching yourself. (If coming together is something you'd like to try, this last option can sometimes help make it work.) Another version of this is to kiss and rub against each other while you each masturbate, or do it side by side. Some couples like to watch each other. Some women also enjoy it if their partner touches them at the same time as they are touching themselves; you might enjoy the feeling of your partners fingers gently moving in and around your vagina while you bring yourself by orgasm by sliding your fingers over your clitoris and labia, or you could do it the other way around.

How we like to be touched varies. There are, you might say, different strokes for different folks, at different times. You might like your partner to touch your pubic hair, brushing against your vaginal lips with a soft stroking motion before moving gradually to other areas, such as the clitoris and the vagina. The clitoris is especially sensitive and is the source of a woman's orgasm. But too much pressure, too soon, can be painful or irritating, so try starting off softly and slowly, gradually increasing the stimulation. Some women, on the other hand, enjoy a firm, sustained rubbing action. You can alter the speed and pressure, and vary the type of movement, depending on what feels good.

82

You might like your partner to move their
fingers round and round in a circle or at other
times to go up and down or side to side. Your
partner could use one or more fingers or the flat
of their hand. You could try different positions:
on your back, lying or sitting facing each other,
on your stomach, standing up or with your
partner lying or sitting behind you – like
spoons. Build up your arousal by letting your
partner's fingers alternate between caressing
your lips and the area around the entrance to
the vagina, and stroking your clitoris. What
does it feel like if they rub the mons pubis or
move the vaginal lips back and forth?
Sometimes it can be more satisfying to touch
the tissues surrounding the clitoris, especially
the area just in front of it, rather than the clitoris
itself – direct stimulation of the clitoris can be
numbing and uncomfortable. It's also possible
to have orgasms by pressure alone, some
women do this by squeezing their thighs
together or rubbing against their partner's
body.

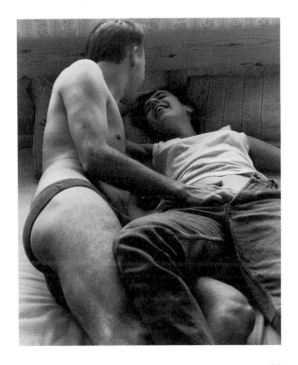

Some women enjoy gentle, teasing stroking just outside the vaginal opening and may also like the feeling of their partner's fingers inside them during lovemaking. One way of doing this is for your partner to slide their finger gently inside your vagina with their hand over your mons pubis so that they can caress your clitoris with their thumb.

Lubricants can help to increase sensation. It doesn't matter how turned on you are, if for some reason you are not wet, it can be hard to enjoy being touched, especially around your clitoris. Water-based lubricants are the safest. (For a full discussion of lubricants and their uses see pages 132–4.)

Tell your partner how you want them to use their hands or, better still, show them what you mean by harder and softer, faster or slower, or where they should touch you, by guiding their hand. You could also show your partner exactly what you like by doing it yourself.

However it's done, there is little or no risk of transmitting HIV during 'mutual masturbation' – the skin is designed to protect you against infection. The only time there might be a risk is if you make a man come by rubbing or stroking his penis and his semen comes into contact with breaks in the skin. Similarly, if a woman is infected and her partner has open sores or cuts on their hands, there could be some risk of infection if they come into contact with her blood or vaginal and cervical secretions. (Transmission is more likely during a woman's period.) Put a plaster over any cuts or scratches or wear disposable rubber gloves if you need to.

If you make love with another woman you might touch her and then touch yourself or use her wetness to lubricate your clitoris and vaginal lips, or vice versa. This can be very arousing but if either of you is infected then there could be some risk of transmission through the moist membranes of the lips and vagina, especially if there are sores or abrasions. Similarly, if either of you have a vaginal infection such as thrush, it too could be passed on by fluid on the fingers. (See also discussion of herpes on page 59.)

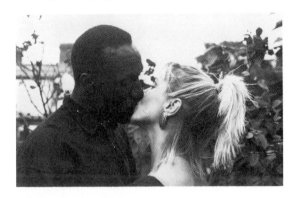

Kissing

Kissing is a very important part of most people's sex-lives. It can communicate desire, love, passion, intimacy, affection and lead to feelings of warmth, tenderness and closeness. It can also be an incredibly exciting and sensual experience which, for many of us, is as much a part of wanting to make love as orgasm itself. Perhaps this is because when we kiss someone we make use of all our senses – you can taste someone's mouth, hear the sound of their breathing, smell their breath and skin, feel their cheek against you, look into their eyes. It's also because the mouth, lips and tongue are all highly sensitive.

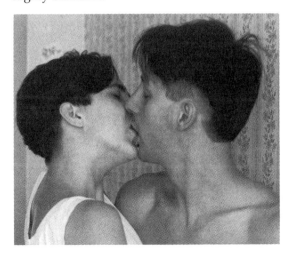

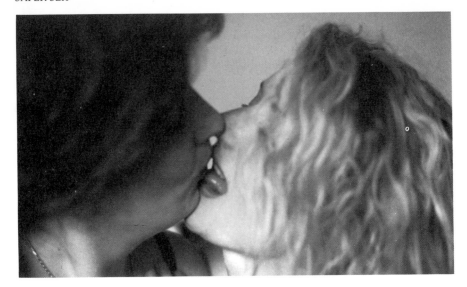

Most experts now believe that it's safe to kiss. While the HIV virus has been found in saliva in small amounts, no one has ever been known to become infected through kissing. The only time when there might theoretically be a slight risk of the virus being passed on is if there are cuts or sores in the mouth and the saliva contains blood.

How we like to be kissed varies from kiss to kiss, and person to person. In some situations we may enjoy passionate, almost continuous kissing during sex, at other times we may prefer to kiss only occasionally or not at all. It can be nice to kiss softly and slowly, with lips closed, or you might enjoy using your tongue to explore the inside of your partner's mouth. This is called French kissing or deep kissing.

Spend time with your partner trying out different ways of kissing. Touch the tips of your tongues together. Slide your tongue over your partner's teeth and inside their lips. What do they taste of? Move your tongue in and out of their mouth. Get your partner to use their mouth to explore your lips. Suck your partner's tongue. Lick each other's lips. Vary the pressure against each other's mouths. It can be a turn on to kiss fleetingly, brushing against each other's lips, as well as more firmly. Try kissing your partner at the same time as playing with their lips with your fingers. Look at each other whilst you kiss. Wet your fingers and moisten their lips. (But remember that if you use vaginal juices to do this the risk is similar to that of cunnilingus – see page 98.) Put some wine in your mouth and pass it from your mouth to theirs. Use your imagination and enjoy it!

Kissing needn't just be restricted to mouths – you can use your mouth to enjoy sex by sucking and kissing each other's bodies. Providing there are no breaks in the skin that could result in exposure to blood, body kissing carries little or no risk of transmission of HIV or other infections. Nibbling on ear lobes, sucking toes and fingers, kissing necks or inner thighs, caressing backs with your tongue, licking armpits, tongueing behind the knees or inside arms, are all activities that are safe and sexy! Biting each other's bodies, including giving one another lovebites, will not transmit the virus as long as you do not draw blood and the same applies to scratching. (Be careful of long or ragged fingernails!)

Body kissing

The body is your oyster. Why not take the time with your partner to discover where, and how, you like being kissed the best.

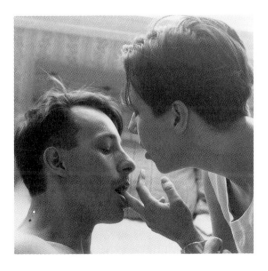

87

Breast kissing

Sucking on nipples is also considered safe as long as they are not cracked or bleeding and, in the case of a woman, if she is not breastfeeding. Many women find that having their breasts and nipples kissed is intensely erotic, and some men find it exciting too. Licking, sucking and nibbling can all feel good – vary the rhythm and the amount of pressure to see how it feels. Some women prefer the rapid flicking of a tongue against their nipple, others prefer having their nipples sucked, long and slow. You may have different preferences at different times, and some women only enjoy very gentle kissing of their breasts just before their period, because they are feeling tender. Or you might like light, teasing tongueing on your breast and nipples when you begin making love but as you become more aroused you may prefer more direct, sustained kissing.

There are lots of ways you can incorporate breast kissing into lovemaking. Some women enjoy getting their partner to cup both breasts together so they can suck both nipples at the same time. Try putting something on your nipples for your partner to lick off (honey, diet coke, champagne?!), or touching one breast with fingers while having the other sucked. Not that the pleasure need all be one way. It can be very exciting to feel your partner's nipples harden and become firm in your mouth. The feel and taste of their skin and body can be very erotic too.

Touch

Many people associate sex only with genital touch but by doing this they are missing out on the sexual pleasures that touching other parts of the body can bring. Hugging, cuddling and caressing are entirely safe, massaging each other's bodies can be very sensual and exciting as well as relaxing, and using massage oils can add to the pleasure.

•

Because there were other people in the room all we could do was kiss and stroke each other. It was the most incredible experience; very sexy; very passionate.

•

Take time with your partner to discover where it feels good to be touched. This might be on the palm of your hand, the back of your neck, the top of your buttocks, your breasts or in the small of your back. Explore the *entire* body. Don't just stick to the so-called ero-

88

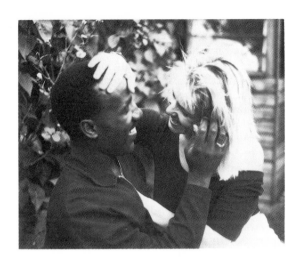

genous zones – vulva, breasts, nipples, penis, scrotum – or you'll be missing out on a lot! If you start by touching your partner, you might caress their cheek, running your fingers firmly and slowly through their hair and over their scalp. Gently stroke their ears and the skin underneath their chin. Bury your face in their hair and enjoy the smell and the texture of it (the pleasures of playing with hair are often underestimated). When they are ready, move on to a different part of their body – you might slide your fingers in and out of their fingers and toes or, using a hard stroking motion, massage their back, pressing your thumbs and fingers up and down their spine and across their buttocks. Lots of people enjoy having their bottom held during sex and are excited by being gripped so that their buttocks are slightly parted. Others like their hips and bottom to be stroked more gently and enjoy a light feathery touch, round and round, just at the top of the cleft in their bottom. Alternatively, get your partner to slowly stroke your abdomen and pubic hair. What does it feel like if they put their finger in your navel? See if you enjoy it if they gently nibble your shoulders and the back of your neck. Rest your hands on your partner's inner thigh, moving your palms down their legs to their ankles. Give them a foot massage, pres-

•

I like being touched all over my body, in different ways.

•

What I really enjoy is for my partner to kiss the back of my neck, while stroking the rest of my back with his fingers.

•

I love having my fingers sucked and a long lick all the way up my arm.

•

sing your thumbs into the spot below the ball of the foot and stroking between their toes.

Experiment with different kinds of touch. You can safely rub, stroke, massage, knead, tickle, brush against, squeeze and gently scratch. You can use your fingertips, thumbs, the palm or the side of your hand, and your knuckles. Stroking can be long and slow, round and round, it can be a tap with a fingertip or it can be short and fleeting. Why not vary the speed and pressure and see what difference that makes. Get your partner to move their finger tips over your body so lightly that they hardly don't touch your skin. When they get to a part that feels especially good tell them to increase the pace and pressure. Try moving your hands in different ways.

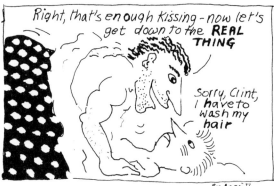

Don't think of this as 'foreplay'. This kind of touch is extremely pleasurable in itself, you don't need to have an orgasm to enjoy it – although you can! Some women come by squeezing their thighs together or by having their breasts and nipples kissed and stroked. Remember that if you or your partner do come, then holding and caressing each other afterwards is an important part of the total experience of sex.

Body rubbing   As well as using your hands and fingertips to stroke and touch each other, you can touch with your chest, arms, breasts, lips, tongue, eyelashes – your whole body in fact. Getting sexual pleasure from rubbing against someone or something is called frottage. Rubbing against each other's bodies can make you feel really close and intimate, and very passionate. A woman may arouse herself and reach orgasm by rubbing her clitoris against her partner's arm, thigh or pubic mound. Men can have orgasms this way too, by rubbing their penis between a woman's breasts, thighs, armpits or against her body. When two women lie on top of each other, or on their sides, and rub against each other it's called tribadism. As long as there are no cuts or breaks in the skin this is safe. Remember that putting a plaster on cuts or open sores will reduce the risk of transmission.

If your partner is a woman, you might enjoy rubbing your vagina against hers (this is sometimes called scissors, because of the position you get into). This may allow transmission of some vaginal infections such as herpes, trichomoniasis and thrush. As vaginal fluids may be exchanged, there could also be a theoretical risk of HIV transmission if one woman was infected and her partner had cuts or abrasions on her genitals, which could allow the virus to get into her bloodstream.

Breasts and nipples

Some women enjoy their breasts being touched a great deal during lovemaking; others don't like their breasts and nipples to be stimulated until they are very aroused and near to orgasm. How responsive our breasts are to touch can also vary at different times, for instance depending on what time of the month it is. Here are some suggestions for ways which you can stimulate your own breasts or your partner's breasts or chest (or vice versa!).

Rest your hands on each breast and slowly circle your thumbs outwards and then back towards the nipple, but don't touch it. Begin with very light movement, hardly touching the skin, and steadily increase the pressure. Using the fingers and thumbs, as well as the palms of the hands, knead each breast slowly and firmly. Cup your hands slightly so that your palm slides over the nipple. Rest your fingertips lightly on the darker skin of the areola and brush the tip of the nipple, slowly at first, then

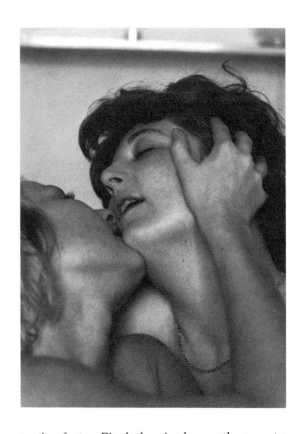

getting faster. Pinch the nipples gently, one at a time and then both together. Flick fingers back and forth across them. With your fingertips, move in circles round and round on the nipple ends, vary the speed and pressure. Roll each nipple between your thumb and forefinger, squeezing gently and then, if it feels good, more firmly. It can be very exciting to touch each other's nipples at the same time; you could also do this with one hand while touching other parts of the body with the other. Some people find it especially arousing to have their nipples stimulated at the same time as their clitoris or penis. Be creative in discovering the different feelings associated with different kinds of touch and which is most arousing. Don't just use hands and fingers; breasts can be stimulated using different parts of the body – mouth, tongue, lips, chest, hair.

Rubbing your breasts against your partner's body is another safe way of expressing yourself sexually, some people like burying their face and nuzzling while others enjoy it if their partner sits above them and touches their face with their breasts and nipples. Rub breasts together or rub yours against your partner's genitals – this is safe assuming you don't have cracked and bleeding nipples.

You could use oil or body lotions, this way hands slide more easily over skin, and bodies against each other, heightening sensation. You can also play with lubricants in this way. (It's important to remember that oil-based lubricants and lotions might perish rubber if they come into contact with condoms, diaphragms or latex barriers. See page 132 for a fuller discussion.) This includes playing with your own or your partner's natural lubrication. For example, you might enjoy smelling and tasting vaginal secretions on your own or your partner's fingers, licking it off their nipples or having them do that for you, but if you do, the risk is similar for cunnilingus (see page 98). Certain foods and drinks may also be fun and safe to play with. Try drinking wine from your partner's navel! Chocaholics may enjoy putting chocolate whip in swirls around their partner's nipples, or at the base of their spine, and licking it off. Simply adapt the recipe according to taste!

In addition to using creams, oils and lubricants, you can experiment with touching and exploring each other's bodies in the bath or the shower. Use your hands or a sponge to make your bodies all wet and soapy. Splash out and make it luxurious – there are lots of nice smelling bath oils, soaps and shower gels to choose from. Discover how rubbing against one another when your bodies are wet and slippery is different to touching dry skin. Have fun wetting each other. Pour water over your hair, backs and shoulders, or use the shower head to spray water on different parts of the body. Does it excite you and make your skin tingle if you increase the pressure? Some women find they

In at the deep end

can have orgasms with a jet of water directed at their clitoris. (If you are having a bath together, open your legs and get your partner to make waves that lap against your vaginal lips and clitoris.) Men can also find it very erotic to feel water pressure from the bath taps or the shower hose against their penis and testicles.

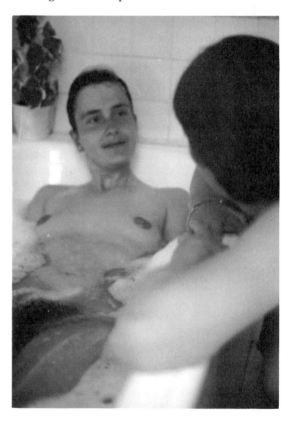

Sex toys   You can also use, among other things, feathers, vibrators, dildoes and massage gloves to stimulate each other's bodies. Vibrators give out consistent, pulsating vibrations and can be used to produce pleasurable sensations all over the body. You can buy vibrators by mail order or in certain shops, and body massagers, which can be used for sex, can be purchased in large chemists. They come in a variety of sizes, shapes and styles. Some are battery operated, others, like the Hitachi Magic Wand body mas-

94

sager, plug into the mains (these are safe as long as you keep them away from water!). Something else to consider is whether or not you can vary the speed. Many women prefer to start off with low vibrations, gradually building up the intensity as they become more aroused. Without any control at your fingertips the experience may be more numbing than ecstatic! If you find even the lowest speed too much too soon, try feeling the vibration through your pants or wrapping the vibrator in something to soften the sensation.

Some women find it very easy to have an orgasm by holding a vibrator against their clitoris, others prefer to insert the vibrator into the vagina and move it slowly in and out. (A man may also enjoy being stimulated with a vibrator, especially around the sensitive tip of his penis.) Be careful putting vibrators into the vagina, or rectum, as they are usually made of hard plastic and it is very easy to damage the delicate tissue. Touch, whether it is by fingers alone or by a 'sex toy', needs to be done with sensitivity and that's as much a part of safer sex as anything else.

I'd really like to try using a vibrator, but I'm afraid I'll become hooked!

You don't have to be scared that you'll become addicted to the vibrator or that you won't be able to enjoy sex again without it. Sex isn't like some kind of energy that, once it's used up, is all gone. Sexual desire comes, and it goes, according to how we feel. The likelihood is that by learning more about how your body works you'll be better able to know what to suggest to a partner during lovemaking. And the better they are at responding to what you like, the more you are going to want to make love. You might also want to add to your safer sex options by using a vibrator with your partner.

Sharing vibrators or dildoes (phallic-shaped objects, usually made of rubber) with your partner is safe as long as they don't come into contact with blood, faeces, cervical or vaginal secretions or semen. If they do there may be a

95

risk of infection with the HIV virus or other sexually transmitted diseases. You can reduce the risk by using a condom over the vibrator or dildo you are sharing, but be sure to use a fresh condom each time you transfer it from one person to another. Alternatively, you can wash the vibrator or dildo in very hot soapy water, or clean your sex toys using household bleach, diluted to one part bleach to ten parts water. (Make sure all the bleach solution is thoroughly washed off before you use it again.) The other golden rule for safer sex is don't use a vibrator or a dildo in someone's anus, or your own, and then put it inside your vagina. It can cause an infection.

Sex toys may be 'home-made', you can use a variety of objects to stimulate the clitoris, vagina and rectum – including candles, cucumbers, carrots and courgettes – make sure that they are clean and/or put a condom on. (Don't be tempted to put bottles in the vagina or rectum, it's dangerous; they could break or create a vacuum and get stuck.) Similarly, some women enjoy pressing their clitoris against other things – from a washing machine to a pillow! By all means experiment (safely, of course), but remember that a lot of sex toys are designed to make money rather than love. Vibrating dildoes with 'clit ticklers', cock-rings, condoms with Mickey Mouse on the end, may make you laugh but that may be the extent of the fun you and your partner get from them. The best sex toy is your body.

Come to your senses   Touch is a very important part of safer sex. We should not, however, ignore the other senses and the part they can play in making sex both exciting and safer. Looking at our partner, and getting to know their body by sight as well as by touch, can be a very powerful sexual experience. The tastes and smells of our bodies can also be intensely erotic, even the smell of a certain perfume or aftershave can be arousing. Listening to the sound of your partner's breathing, and the sounds they make as you touch them, can be a real thrill. And talking to each other while making love can be very exciting.

You don't necessarily have to be together to do this – there is always telephone sex! You can turn each other on by talking to each other on the phone at the same time as you are touching yourself or give each other a verbal massage, describing in detail how you would like to touch one another. Obviously this has to be a two-way game – otherwise it's just an abusive phone-call.

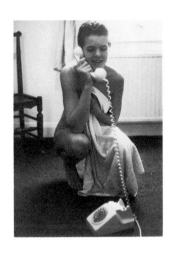

As well as sounds, smells and tastes, thoughts and memories can make you feel very sexual. Reading a letter from your lover, remembering a time when you made love very passionately, thinking of a scene from a movie, imagining having sex with someone you desire, are all things that can be arousing. You can also use your mind to be sexually creative – there's no need always to make love in the same place, be it in the back of a car or the bedroom. A change of scenery – in front of the TV, in the shower, by a roaring fire, out of doors – can add to your safer sex options. Be varied! People can make love in the dark, with dim lighting or in broad daylight. Some people like to have background music playing, others enjoy sex in the bath. You can touch each other with clothes on or off, enjoy dressing and undressing each other. You can be imaginative about when you make love. If you've got into the habit of always making love on Sunday mornings, try tea-time on Thursdays instead! Another way of broadening your safer sex options is to try doing the things you like in different positions.

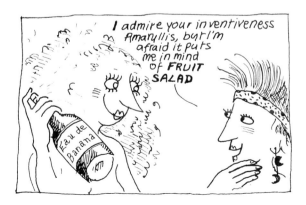

Oral sex   Oral sex is when someone uses their mouth and tongue to kiss, lick or suck their partner's genitals. When a woman is stimulated in this way it is called cunnilingus. There are a variety of different ways of having oral sex that can be both extremely pleasurable and highly arousing. Some women enjoy light, darting tongue movements around the clitoris, others enjoy more rapid, focused licking, or having their clitoris sucked gently. The pleasure need not be all one way. To smell and taste the warm moistness of a woman's clitoris and vaginal lips can be a real turn on for her partner. Other techniques you might enjoy with your partner are being kissed and licked while they are stimulating your vagina and the area just outside it with their fingers or having their tongue move in and out of your vagina, and having them stroke your clitoris with their fingers while they use their mouth to stimulate other parts of your genitals.

When a woman (or man) licks, kisses or sucks a man's penis it is called fellatio. As with cunnilingus, the pressure, speed and movement can be varied for different kinds of sensation. Oral sex can be done with one person stimulating their partner, or you might want to do it to each other at the same time. When a couple lie side-by-side or on top of one another and lick and suck each other off it is called 69 or soixante-neuf. You might both enjoy this, but is it safe?

You can't get pregnant by having oral sex but most sexually transmitted diseases, including gonorrhoea and herpes, can be passed on this way. Whether the HIV virus can be transmitted during oral sex is not clear. Studies suggest that transmission is difficult if you have a healthy mouth because HIV is killed by acids in the stomach. However, although it is probably unlikely, there may be some risk in going down on someone if you have bleeding gums or cuts and sores in and around your mouth. During fellatio, for example, the virus might be passed on in semen or pre-cum, if the man is infected. Using a condom will reduce the risk to you if you have oral sex with a man. Because

98

lubricated condoms don't taste very nice, you may prefer to use the unlubricated kind. Condoms, their various qualities and how to use them, are discussed in the following chapter.

Is it safe for me to have oral sex with my boyfriend if he doesn't come in my mouth?
A man's pre-cum, which is secreted from the penis before ejaculation, may contain the virus. But if you have a healthy mouth you should not be at risk.

There is probably little or no risk of HIV infection to the man because, although the virus has been isolated in saliva, there is no evidence that it can be transmitted by kissing, licking or sucking. The only time such activities might theoretically carry a risk is if the saliva contained blood. Similarly there is little or no risk to the woman who is enjoying having her clitoris and vagina kissed and caressed by someone's mouth during cunnilingus. (But you can get herpes this way, see page 59.) Where there is a risk, it is for the person doing it: the vaginal and cervical secretions as well as the menstrual blood of women infected with HIV may contain the virus. If this person has bleeding gums, mouth ulcers or any cuts or abrasions in the mouth, the virus may be able to get into the bloodstream. But if you have a normal, healthy mouth, the virus will not be able to get into the bloodstream.

One way of reducing the risk of HIV infection and, most importantly STDs, is to use a latex barrier or, as it is sometimes called, a dental dam. These are sheets of thin rubber about five inches square, originally designed for use in dental surgery, which you place over the vulva to prevent the virus from being transmitted. Some people use cling film or saran wrap but these have not been tested for safety and it's questionable how well they protect. Latex barriers come in many sizes, colours, tastes (you can even get mint!) and thicknesses. You can buy them from surgical and dental supply companies and some mail order firms now sell them. Make sure you rinse latex barriers first: if they have been treated with talcum powder this could irritate the vagina. Putting some water-based lubricant between the vulva and the barrier will increase sensation and, if it contains nonoxynol-9, will add another layer of protection against HIV. As nonoxynol-9 irritates some women, you should test any product containing it on the side of your wrist before using it for sex. If you do get an allergic reaction try using a different brand (see page 128).

Latex barriers don't have to spoil your enjoyment of oral sex. Many women who've used them not only find it as easy to come as before during cunnilingus but they find that it brings new fun and excitement to sex. Try stretching a dam over your partner's nipples and suck them in a bubble of rubber. How does it feel when they do this over your clitoris?

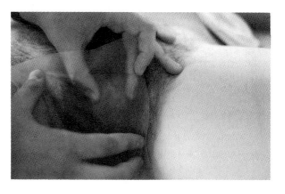

A problem some people find with latex barriers is that it can be difficult to hold them in place whilst making love. One solution is to make a pair of safe sex pants. Cut the gusset out of a pair of pants and fit a barrier in its place. That way the barrier stays put and hands are free to touch and explore in other ways. Another, less aesthetic, suggestion is to wear the barrier as a mask by attaching elastic ties. You could also cut a condom in half and use that instead of a latex barrier – they have the advantage of being easier to buy and are usually thinner and more transparent. As before, unlubricated condoms are more pleasant for using during oral sex because they taste much better than lubricated ones.

Another way of reducing risk is to avoid having oral sex while a woman is having her period and, because there may be some blood mixed with vaginal secretions, immediately before and after.

Some people enjoy it if their partner uses their mouth and tongue to stimulate the area around the anus. This is known as analingus or 'rimming'. As there are a lot of germs which live inside the anus there are certain health risks, including hepatitis, associated with this. HIV has not been shown to be transmitted by faeces but there could be a risk if they contain blood. As with cunnilingus and fellatio, the risk is to the person doing the kissing or licking, especially if they have sores or cuts in the mouth. It is safest to avoid rimming but if you do have oral-anal sex then use a latex barrier between the mouth and the anus to reduce the risk of transmission of STDs and hepatitis.

'Scat', sex which involves defecation, carries similar health risks, especially if faeces come into contact with mucous membranes or nicks or sores on the skin. Similar considerations apply to 'watersports' or 'golden showers' which refer to sex involving urine (urinating on or in someone). There is no evidence of HIV definitely being transmitted this way, however, as there may be blood cells which can transmit the virus in urine, it is safest to avoid urine coming into direct contact with the rectum, vagina or any cuts or abrasions on the skin or in the mouth. Similarly, S/M (sado-masochistic) activities which cause bleeding are not safe. Any kind of sexual behaviour that breaks the skin or draws blood carries a risk of HIV transmission, and relationships that associate sex with pain and humiliation can be psychologically unsafe.

Fantasies can be a way of getting into the right mood for masturbation or having sex with someone or they can be enjoyed simply for themselves. They can be elaborately scripted with a cast of characters and a detailed plot or

Sexual fantasies

101

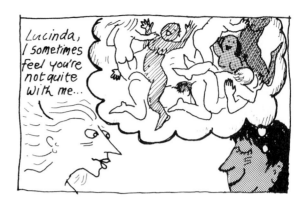

brief flashes of events or expressions which can 'trigger' sexual excitement. What you think about when you fantasize can range from remembering past sexual experiences, imagining things you've never done, daydreaming about sex with different partners, focusing on a specific image – a passionate kiss, a certain phrase, a particular smell – or making love with someone you find sexually attractive.

When they make us feel positive, fantasies are an important part of safer sex. Unfortunately, not all of our fantasies may be like this. Some can be unpleasant or frightening: it's not uncommon for women to have sexual fantasies in which they imagine they are being forced into having sex. Although they find them exciting at the time, women who have fantasies involving violence or domination sometimes say that afterwards they feel troubled. Given the very real threat of sexual violence most women fear, to eroticize such acts as part of lovemaking can be to take certain risks with our minds, if not our bodies. Fantasies which conflict with our feelings and values can be, ultimately, psychologically unsafe. Sometimes fantasies are not healthy for other reasons. Some people use fantasy as an escape from reality, or as a way of distancing themselves from their partner rather than facing up to the problems in their relationship. If you have fantasies that are upsetting, you could work out a new fantasy for yourself that you feel you can accept.

Most women and men fantasize when they masturbate. Some people also do this when they are having sex with a partner, and some women use fantasies to help them reach orgasm. You might decide you want to share sexual fantasies with your partner and this is safe, unless you find listening to each other's fantasies upsetting or threatening. Sometimes shared fantasy can provoke feelings of jealousy or insecurity and if that's the case then either don't share your fantasies, or talk through your fears and insecurities beforehand.

Having learnt that your partner is turned on by a particular fantasy, you might wonder if they want to try it. If you do agree to act it out – make sure that it's a safer sex fantasy, and that you don't feel scared or alienated by it.

You can incorporate fantasy into your lovemaking in other ways. Pretend that you are both lying on a Greek beach with the warm sun on your face, a smell of lemons in the air and the distant sound of the sea against the shore, that you are rolling naked amongst leaves in the middle of a wood or that you have just met, and relive some of your more romantic and passionate memories. Or invent new ones! You could pretend to be a new fantasy lover, and describe yourself and what kind of things turn you on.

This chapter has been about ways of being sexual that won't get you pregnant and involve little or no risk of transmitting HIV and other infections. There are many other safer sex options that could have been mentioned, but that's not really the point. Safer sex isn't just about reeling off a list of things you can do. Much more than that, safer sex is about using the most important sexual organ of the body – our brain. It's about being creative in thinking about ways of making love safely and using your imagination to put your ideas into practice. It's also about the kind of relationships we have with other people, especially around issues like power, trust and responsibility and not feeling pressurised or intimidated into having sex by our partners.

Sex can't be divorced from how we feel; it's

I'm being kissed passionately while two women are sucking my nipples and another is licking my clitoris.

One of my favourite fantasies is about watching my lover make love with someone else.

A man lies down next to me on the beach. He doesn't say anything and then suddenly he is touching me and we are making love. Part of the excitement is knowing that at any time someone might come along and find us.

Safer relationships

CAN YOU PASS THE SAFER-SEX TEST?

Here is a list of things that you might do or like to do (or might be talked into). It groups the safest activities at the beginning and ends with the least safe, so you can see at a glance whether you're practising safer sex. Go through it, perhaps with your partner.

- ☐ Being creative about when and where you make love
- ☐ Massage
- ☐ Touching a woman or man's chest and nipples
- ☐ Kissing
- ☐ Sensual bathing
- ☐ Body to body rubbing
- ☐ Sharing fantasies
- ☐ Body kissing
- ☐ Mutual masturbation
- ☐ Putting fingers in vagina
- ☐ Putting fingers in anus
- ☐ Sucking/licking a woman's genitals using a latex barrier
- ☐ Sucking a man's penis with a condom
- ☐ Rimming
- ☐ Sucking/licking a woman's genitals
- ☐ Sucking a man's penis
- ☐ Sharing sex toys
- ☐ Vaginal intercourse with a condom and spermicide
- ☐ Anal intercourse using a condom and lubricant
- ☐ Fisting
- ☐ Vaginal intercourse
- ☐ Anal intercourse

how we feel about someone that determines whether what you do together is exciting and enjoyable or unerotic and unsafe. Safer sex means being able to say what we want and say no to what we don't want. If you are able to do this with your sexual partners, great! But if, like some women, you are in a relationship where the responsibility for discussing safer sex is not shared equally, or you cannot assert your own needs, you may be at risk in more ways than one. These and other issues to do with negotiating safer sex are discussed later in Chapter 5.

CHAPTER FOUR

RISK
REDUCTION

How you feel about safer sex will depend on your attitudes towards sex. What does sex mean to you? To what extent is it an important part of your life and how you see yourself? What do you most enjoy doing? The level of risk reduction you are willing to take is likely to depend on the answers to these and similar kinds of questions. It will be a decision based on your individual lifestyle and desires. If you enjoy the feeling of a penis, fingers or some other object inside you during lovemaking then you need to know about ways of making your sex-life safer.

In this chapter, we will look at how to make penetrative sex – especially vaginal and anal intercourse – safer.

What's the difference between penetrative sex and sexual intercourse?
Sex which involves inserting a penis into the vagina or anus is called sexual intercourse or, to be more precise, vaginal intercourse and anal intercourse. Penetrative sex includes intercourse but it also refers to sex which involves putting fingers, sex-toys or some other object inside the vagina or anus of another person. (Some might also want to argue that fellatio – sucking on a man's penis – is penetrative sex.) Clearly it is only possible for a woman to have

intercourse with a man but she could have penetrative sex with a woman or penetrate a man's anus.

There are lots of reasons why vaginal intercourse can be unsafe. Unless you are using a reliable method of contraception you will be at risk of getting pregnant. Even then, no method of birth control is 100% effective and while they may make sex safer, some contraceptives can put women's health at risk in other ways. Sexually transmitted infections are spread through vaginal intercourse and it seems there is a link with cervical cancer. It also carries a high degree of risk of infection with HIV, especially if the man does not wear a condom. Ways of reducing the risk of unplanned pregnancy and other sexually transmitted infections besides HIV have already been discussed in Chapter 2. How can you protect yourself from HIV infection and the possibility of developing AIDS?

The HIV virus can be passed on in blood, semen or vaginal or cervical secretions. This means that if a woman engages in sexual activity with a man that allows his blood or semen to get into her body, she will be at risk if he has the virus. During intercourse, the virus might enter your bloodstream through small cuts or tears in the vagina which normally occur as a result of friction and usually go unnoticed. Very occasionally a woman may have vaginal lacerations because of her IUD, or because douching before or after sex can also cause the vagina to tear and bleed. And remember, douching is also ineffective as a way of preventing pregnancy since sperm can swim through the cervix before you've had chance to use it. Douching after vaginal intercourse washes away bacteria which normally help prevent infection, and as well as putting you at greater risk of contracting HIV and vaginal infections, such as thrush, it can also force harmful bacteria up into the uterus, putting you at risk of pelvic inflammatory disease.

Another way the HIV virus might pass into a woman's bloodstream is by being absorbed through the vaginal walls. Cuts or sores on a woman's genitals, and ulcerations of the cervix, may also be a possible route of infection. So, women who have other sexually transmitted diseases, such as herpes and gonorrhoea, may be at greater risk of infection with HIV.

The virus is found in the vaginal and cervical secretions and menstrual blood of HIV-infected women, which is why there is greater risk to the man if intercourse takes place during a woman's period. In men, the virus might enter the bloodstream through the moist membrane lining the entrance to the urethra (the small opening at the tip of the penis), and in uncircumcized men it might be possible for the virus to be absorbed through the moist skin which is covered by the foreskin. But it may be passed more easily if there are cuts or sores on his penis, or if he has a dry and inflamed urethra, allowing the virus more direct access to his bloodstream.

Is it safer if the man withdraws before he comes?

Withdrawal is not going to protect you against unplanned pregnancy or infection. Many men produce some secretion from their penis prior to ejaculation and this pre-cum can contain sperm and may allow HIV and other sexually transmitted infections to be passed on via the vagina. (Withdrawal will not reduce the risk to the man of the virus being passed on by vaginal and cervical secretions or blood in the woman's vagina.) The risk to the woman is increased by the fact that she's got to trust the man to pull out in time, and even then it can be difficult to get the timing right. Don't trust to luck, use your condom-sense!

So, when you have vaginal intercourse you can best reduce the risk of infection and pregnancy by using a condom in conjunction with a spermicide and/or lubricant containing nonoxynol-9. Vaginal intercourse with a condom is not completely safe because some people do not use them properly, and they can tear or come off during intercourse.

A further measure of protection is to use a

diaphragm or cervical cap with a spermicidal cream or gel containing nonoxynol-9. These protect the cervix and the uterus but not the vagina and so, by themselves, they are not sufficient protection against infection (though when used properly with a spermicide, caps and diaphragms are a reliable method of birth control).

Although it won't get you pregnant or increase your risk of cervical cancer, sex where a man puts his penis inside your anus is definitely not safer sex. By doing this you run the risk of getting hepatitis B and other sexually transmitted infections, such as rectal gonorrhoea, herpes and syphilis. And it is by having anal intercourse that you are at most risk of becoming infected with HIV.

Anal intercourse

Anal intercourse is often thought of as something only gay men do. This is evident in the way we often describe it as homosexual intercourse and vaginal intercourse as heterosexual intercourse. The danger with this is that, besides stereotyping gay-male relationships, a man and a woman may think that they are not at risk if they have anal intercourse because what they do is not 'homosexual'. To the virus, however, a male anus is no different to a female anus! Women can become infected with HIV through anal as well as vaginal intercourse, although the risk of infection during anal intercourse with an infected partner is probably considerably higher. The lining of the rectum is very delicate and tears easily during anal sex, such breaks or tears can provide a way into the bloodstream for a variety of sexually transmitted infections, including HIV. The virus can also pass into the bloodstream by being absorbed through the walls of the rectum, which are designed to absorb fluids readily and are very thin.

Although the greatest risk is to the person being penetrated during anal intercourse, it is also possible for the virus to be passed on to the man who is penetrating. Unless he uses a condom it's likely that his penis will come into contact with blood and bloody faeces in the rectum. Again if there are cuts or abrasions on his penis or if he has a dry and inflamed urethra, any infected blood from his partner has a way of getting into his own bloodstream.

If you don't want to give up anal intercourse, it's important to reduce the risk of infection as much as possible – your partner should always wear a condom. If the anus is not well lubricated the condom could tear or come off, as well as it being painful, so use a water-based lubricant such as K Y jelly (oil-based lubricants will damage the rubber). Apart from helping to prevent the condom from ripping, the use of a lubricant will help reduce friction and possible damage to the rectal walls. You might use one containing nonoxynol-9 because of its ability to destroy a wide variety of sexually transmitted infections. But it's important to remember that this product has only been tested for vaginal intercourse: it may not be safe to use on the rectum (see page 132).

A lot of people use a douche or enema before they have anal sex as a hygienic measure. However, this may cause small tears and is likely to increase your risk of H I V infection. So, in view of this and what was discussed under vaginal intercourse, do not douche before or after anal or vaginal sex.

Remember that bacteria that are normally present in the anus can cause vaginal infections, so moving from anal intercourse to vaginal intercourse is unsafe. If you and your partner do this use two separate condoms for anal and vaginal penetration.

In case the condom does get damaged, or falls off, it's safer for the man to withdraw his penis before he ejaculates. This does not mean, however, that anal intercourse is safe as long as a man doesn't climax inside you. Always use a condom to reduce the risk of becoming infected with H I V and other sexually transmitted infections. And the same is true for vaginal intercourse.

Vibrators and sex-toys

Other forms of penetrative sex may also involve some risk. For example, vibrators and other sex toys are sometimes used by women as a way of gaining sexual pleasure. This may include putting them in the vagina, which could be risky if you share your sex-toys (see page 96). (You can also pass on herpes or a yeast infection like thrush by sharing a dildo or vibrator.) To reduce the risk of the virus being transmitted from one person to another, clean and dry sex-toys thoroughly between each partner's use. If you don't want to interrupt your lovemaking, put a condom on your vibrator, dildo or your other sex-toys to help reduce the risk of infection if they are shared. Remember, anything that has been inserted into the anus should not be put into the vagina unless it has been thoroughly washed, or use a new condom.

Fingers

Some women enjoy it if their partner stimulates their vagina with their fingers, by sliding them inside and moving them in and out. This is sometimes called 'finger fucking'.

The chances of the HIV virus being passed on by having sex using fingers are very low but if you or your partner have open sores or cuts on your hands, there could be some risk of infection during vaginal – or anal – penetration. (It's also possible to get vaginal infections by inserting fingers in the anus and then in the vagina. If you or your partner do this, wash your hands in between.) Putting fingers into the vagina of a woman while she is menstruating carries more risk. Long or ragged fingernails or jewellery can cause tiny tears in the vagina and rectum which may also lead to bleeding. If you have an open cut or sore on your finger putting on a plaster or, if you have an eczema-like rash, wearing disposable rubber gloves will reduce the risk of the virus being passed on from one person to another via blood or vaginal secretions. Alternatively, you can put a condom on your or your partner's fingers, and using a water-based lubricant will increase your sensation as well as adding a further layer of protection if it contains nonoxynol-9.

Fisting

'Fisting', where one person inserts their hand into the vagina or rectum of another person, is risky for both partners. The partner who is

111

inserting their hand may be exposed to blood and/or vaginal fluids containing HIV, whereas the person being fist-fucked is at risk because the walls of the vagina or rectum are likely to tear, causing bleeding. This makes it very easy for blood from a sore or cut on a person's hand to enter the bloodstream. Fisting can also cause severe internal injuries, as well as increasing the risk of transmission of the HIV virus, if you have intercourse – vaginal or anal – afterwards.

Unless the vagina or anus is well-lubricated putting anything inside it is likely to be painful. If, despite the risks, you engage in fisting, use plenty of water-based lubricant. If it is for use in the vagina choose one that contains nonoxynol-9, which is known to be effective against HIV. It's not clear what effect nonoxynol-9 has on the rectum and whether you should use it for anal sex (see page 132 for a fuller discussion of nonoxynol-9 and lubricants). Using a thin rubber glove (the kind used for internal examinations, not for washing up!) will also reduce the risk of transmission of HIV during anal or vaginal fisting, especially if a person has open cuts, scratches or skin rashes – like eczema – on their hands. Rubber gloves also cause less friction than bare hands and reduce the risk of tears or scratches, but throw the glove away afterwards. Disposable rubber gloves can be bought in most chemists and from medical supply firms.

Condom-sense

Condoms are an important way of making sex safer, they are readily available, free or relatively inexpensive, and, with practice, easy to use. They have no adverse side-effects, apart from the occasional allergic reaction to the rubber or chemicals used in the lubrication, and when they are used *correctly and consistently*, in combination with a spermicide, they are a very effective means of birth control. If they are used properly, condoms can also reduce the risk of the HIV virus being transmitted during vaginal and anal intercourse, and during oral sex. This is because the virus, like sperm, is not able to pass through rubber. Condoms can also help to

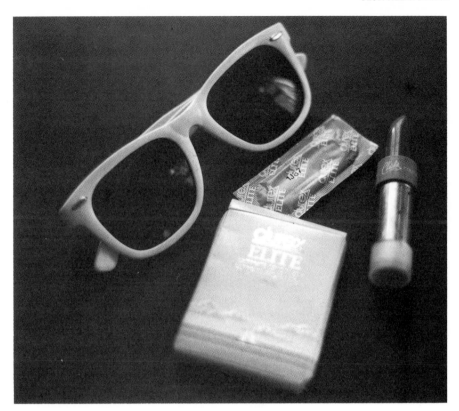

protect you from most other sexually transmitted diseases including gonorrhoea, herpes and chlamydia. They have no health risks, unlike most other contraceptives, and they can also help to prevent cancer of the cervix. Many women also find too that no post-intercourse drippiness is a big advantage!

Condoms are good news but it's important to remember that they do not make sex 100% safe. They have about a 2–15% failure rate in preventing pregnancy (which means that out of 100 couples using the condom *for a year*, about 2–15 women become pregnant), and the protection they give against HIV infection could be lower. A woman can get pregnant only a few days every month, but she is at risk of HIV infection every time she has sexual intercourse with an infected partner.

Why do condoms fail? The main reason that condoms fail is incorrect use. Sometimes the condom is damaged as it is taken out of the packet, or else it is put on or taken off incorrectly. But another reason why condoms don't always prevent disease or pregnancy is that they can break or tear (this is why they must always be used with a spermicide). Usually they break or tear because they are old (always check the sell-by date), because there is air in the condom or because insufficient lubrication or an oil-based lubricant, like Vaseline, is used. Condoms were originally designed for vaginal intercourse and because the anus tends to be drier and tighter, it is more likely that they will tear or come off during anal intercourse, so use plenty of lubrication. Some condoms, such as HT Special and Durex Extra Strong, are much thicker and *may* be less likely to rip if you have anal sex.

Occasionally condoms leak or break because they are poorly made, which is why you should always use brands which have been tested for safety and reliability (see the Buyer's Guide to Condoms on page 120). Another form of risk reduction is for the man to withdraw his penis before he comes. This will decrease the chance of sperm or HIV getting through if the condom should break. You might think of using two condoms instead of one, for extra protection, but this does *not* necessarily make sex safer – the two layers of rubber can rub against each other and burst.

Getting into practice A condom may be worn by a man but that doesn't mean women don't need to know how

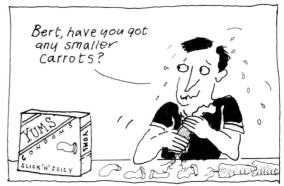

114

to put them on. That's *not* to say that men should rely on women to take responsibility for safe sex – they need to practise too! You'll find your guide to using condoms on page 124. Follow the instructions in the packet carefully and remember that practice makes perfect. You probably weren't very good at tying your shoelaces the first time you tried! It's the same with putting on a condom, you may need to put them on several times before it seems natural and easy. You might want to learn to do this with your partner and if you do, make sure you practice your technique safely and that you've got the hang of putting a condom on before you use one for penetrative or oral sex. You could also practise with a vibrator, cucumber or carrot. If you make a mistake – open another one and try again. See what it feels like when the condom breaks. Men can learn to identify the difference in how it feels by breaking a condom on their penis while masturbating, and so when a condom breaks during intercourse they will know and can withdraw to put on a new one. The more you use condoms, the more experienced you will become and accidents are less likely to occur.

Is there any way to make using condoms less intrusive during sex?
If you are new to condoms you may feel that the whole procedure of unwrapping the packet and rolling the condom on spoils the spontaneity of lovemaking, but this needn't be the case. Putting a condom on can become as easy and as exciting a part of making love as changing positions. If you can't practise with your partner, try putting a condom on a banana or on your fingers. See if you can unroll it with your eyes closed – it might help you avoid putting it on the wrong way if you make love in the dark. You may find that rather than interrupting sex, putting a condom on becomes incorporated into your lovemaking.

I use a diaphragm, surely my partner doesn't need to use a condom?
It's important to be clear why you are using

> **Remember the basics:**
> Put condoms on and take them off properly.
> Always use brands that have been tested for strength and reliability, and which have an expiry date.
> Only used water-based spermicides or lubricants.
> Never use oil-based products.
> Be prepared, willing and able to use them!

condoms. People often confuse contraception and disease prevention. If you want to reduce your risk of infection you should use a condom during intercourse, irrespective of whether or not you are already using some other method of contraception. The diaphragm, the IUD or the pill may be effective in preventing pregnancy but they will not protect you from the HIV virus or most other sexually transmitted diseases.

Concerns about condoms

Another reason why condoms fail to protect against infection and pregnancy is if you don't use them *consistently* – here are some of the reasons people give:

It doesn't feel as good with a condom.
Many men complain that wearing a condom lessens sensation. This is certainly not a good enough reason to put your own or someone else's life at risk. It's also not necessarily true. Condoms can reduce stimulation slightly for both women and men, but nowadays you can get a wide variety of condoms which, while they are strong and tough, are so fine that you barely notice them.

He might lose his erection while he's putting it on.
If it affects a man's erection slightly – don't worry. Don't make the mistake of thinking that once he's got the condom on you must have intercourse immediately, or that he must come. Use as many condoms during sex as you like.

It interrupts sex to have to stop and put them on.
You don't have a bus to catch do you? Sex isn't a non-stop race and, with practice, putting on a condom can be really quick and easy. It can also be fun. You can put the condom on your partner or watch him put it on.

I'd be too embarrassed to buy them.
Maybe you feel a little guilty about planning to have sex? OK, so the fact that you are buying condoms says that you are sexually active –

almost everyone is! At least you are being responsible about it, and it needn't be that difficult. Most chemists and other shops selling condoms display them on the counter so you don't have to ask for them. You can just pop them in your shopping basket along with the rest of your shopping and pay at the checkout. You could also get them free from family planning clinics, buy them from slot machines in toilets or through a mail order firm.

My partner might be offended.
You never know he might be glad that you've raised the subject. But if he does feel insulted, make it clear that by practising safer sex you are both protected. If your partner refuses to wear condoms you could suggest some of the exciting sexual possibilities that do not involve penetration. Or you might decide that you'd rather not have sex with him at all. If you have sex without a condom just to please your partner it won't do much for your self-esteem and it may put your health at risk. Are you willing to take that risk?

Q: Which of these blokes has an STD?

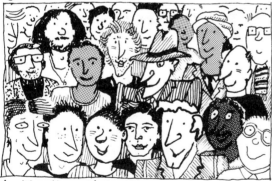

A: Yep, it could be any one of em!

I don't really need them.
It's easy to believe someone you really like and want to go to bed with is not the kind of person who has an infection, but *how are you going to know?* You can't tell simply from looking at someone whether or not they are infected with

something and they might not tell you if they injected drugs and shared needles or took other risks before they met you. If either you or your partner have had unsafe sex with other partners, or shared equipment to inject drugs, it is advisable to use condoms if you have intercourse, especially if there is a possibility that one of you had sex with someone who may have been infected with the HIV virus. You might also want to use them, in combination with a spermicide, as a form of contraception that has no health risks.

I want sex to be spontaneous.
The answer is simple: Be Prepared! If you usually make love in bed, then have condoms handy. One woman I know keeps them in a jewellery box on her dressing table. Similarly, keep a supply of condoms in the car, the front room, anywhere you might have sex. And when you go out on a date with someone you want to have sex with, take them with you, just in case you decide to have intercourse and he's run out.

We've been together for 3 years. How can I explain suddenly wanting to use condoms to my partner?
Sometimes it can seem more difficult to raise the subject of safer sex with someone you know very well than with a new partner. You may have got into the habit of not talking about sex and just 'doing it' or you may feel that to suggest using condoms would be to imply that one of you is having an affair. One way of introducing the idea of using condoms is to talk about general health concerns, or how you can make sex more exciting. How to negotiate safer sex is discussed more fully in Chapter 5.

I've been practising safer sex with my partner for some time, but now I've decided I want to become pregnant. I don't want to put myself at risk of HIV infection. What should I do?
There are no simple answers to this particular question. One possibility is to carefully consider, with your partner, whether or not you

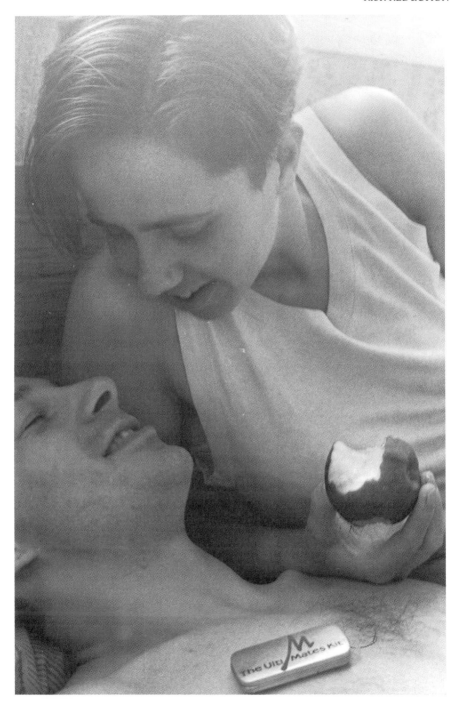

BUYER'S GUIDE TO CONDOMS

BRAND	COUNTRY OF MANUFACTURE	COLOUR	SURFACE	SHAPE	TEAT-ENDED
Aegis Snugfit	W Germany	beige	smooth	plain	no
Aegis Bigboy	W Germany	beige	smooth	plain	no
Duet Supersafe Fully Shaped	W Germany	beige	smooth	contoured	yes
Duet Supersafe Ultra Thin	W Germany	beige	smooth	plain	yes
*Duet Supersafe Ribbed	W Germany	beige	ribbed	contoured	yes
*Duet Supersafe Studded	W Germany	beige	studded	plain	yes
Durex Allergy	UK	beige	smooth	plain	yes
Durex Arouser	UK	pink	ribbed	plain	yes
Durex Black Shadow	UK	black	smooth	plain	yes
Durex Elite	UK	beige	smooth	plain	yes
Durex Extra Strong	UK	beige	smooth	plain	yes
Durex Fetherlite	UK	pink	smooth	plain	yes
Durex Fiesta	UK	various	smooth	plain	yes
Durex Gold	UK	gold	smooth	plain	no
Durex Gossamer	UK	beige	smooth	plain	yes
Durex Nu-form Extra Safe	UK	pink	smooth	contoured	yes
HT Special	W Germany	beige	smooth	plain	yes
Jiffi Gold	not stated	beige	smooth	contoured	yes
Mates	US	beige	smooth	contoured	yes
Mentor	US	beige	smooth	plain	yes
Premex Coral Superfine Dry	UK	pink	smooth	plain	yes
Prime	US	beige	smooth	contoured	yes
*Protex Pro Form	Korea	coral	smooth	plain	yes
Red Stripe	Japan	beige	smooth	plain	no
Ribbed Mates	US	beige	ribbed	plain	yes
Superstrong Mates	US	beige	smooth	plain	yes

KITEMARK	LUBRICANT	NONOXYNOL-9	THICKNESS (mm)	TESTED FOR FREEDOM FROM HOLES	TESTED FOR STRENGTH
no	L	no	0.05	pass	pass
no	DRY	no	0.06	pass	pass
no	SL	no	0.06	pass	pass
no	SL	no	0.05	pass	pass
no	SL	no	0.06	fail	fail
no	SL	no	0.06	fail	fail
yes	L	no	0.05	pass	pass
yes	L	no	0.06	pass	pass
yes	L	no	0.05	pass	pass
yes	SL	yes	0.05	pass	pass
yes	SL	yes	0.1	pass	extra strong
yes	L	no	0.05	pass	pass
yes	L	no	0.05	pass	pass
yes	SL	yes	0.05	pass	pass
yes	L	no	0.05	pass	pass
yes	SL	yes	0.05	pass	pass
no	L	no	0.09	pass	extra strong
no	SL	yes	0.05	pass	pass
yes	SL	yes	0.05	pass	pass
no	L	no	0.05	pass	pass
no	DRY	no	0.05	pass	pass
no	SL	yes	0.07	pass	pass
no	L	no	0.07	fail	pass
no	L	no	0.06	pass	pass
yes	SL	yes	0.06	pass	pass
–	SL	yes	0.1	pass	extra strong

N.B.: L=Lubricant. SL=Spermicidal Lubricant.

*Condoms that are not recommended for safe sex

need to take the HIV antibody test. For reasons that have already been discussed (see page 71) you should only take the test after a full discussion of what the test's results mean and how they could affect your life. If your partner is infected, you could decide to have a child by artificial insemination using a donor whose sperm is clear. Nowadays clinics offering artificial insemination screen donors for HIV infection, but of course this needs a great deal of thought and discussion.

Choosing a condom

Although it is men who wear condoms, women need to know about them too. After all, you are on the receiving end of the condom, it's your body the condom is going into.

There are many different kinds of condoms to choose from. You can get smooth or ribbed ones, dry or lubricated, sensitive or extra-sensitive, straight or shaped, with a teat at the tip or plain-ended. They come in different thicknesses, shapes, sizes, colours, and flavours. And the best way of deciding which one suits you and your partner is to shop around. Like trying on shoes or clothes, buy some different brands, and experiment to find out which you prefer. You can get them from chemists, slot machines in toilets, garages, supermarkets, and by mail order. (Look in the personal column of magazines and newspapers for addresses of companies that do a postal delivery.) Condoms are also available free, to both men and women, from family planning clinics, although they are unlikely to offer a wide choice of brands and styles.

When you are picking the condom that's right for you the main thing is to determine what you like, what you don't like and how effective it is in reducing risk. Lubricated condoms – some are coated with a lubricating spermicide containing nonoxynol-9 – do not break as easily as unlubricated ones. Another way of reducing the risk of the condom breaking is to use a strong condom. More important than thickness is the age of the condom and the way it is handled. Don't store condoms near heat (for example near a radiator) or in strong sunlight as the rubber will deteriorate. Don't test condoms before you use them, by blowing them up or stretching them, and don't use old condoms – check the expiry date on the packet. If it is past the use-by date, or hasn't got one, throw it away. In Britain, you should also look on the packet for the British Standard Institute Kitemark. This means that the condom has passed tests for strength and reliability in vaginal intercourse. They are not guaranteed for anal intercourse but *providing* you use sufficient lubrication, there may be no greater risk of tearing than with vaginal intercourse.

Condoms which do not carry the Kitemark may not be safe to use for vaginal or anal intercourse but this does not mean that all condoms without a Kitemark are unsafe. Some, such as Prime and HT Special, may have passed very strict tests in their country of origin and be a reliable brand to use but don't carry a Kitemark because they are imported. Hopefully there will soon be an internationally agreed standard which will make it much easier to know which imported brands are safe to use, and which aren't.

The taste and smell of the condom is very important for oral sex. Some condoms taste appalling because of their lubricants or the taste of the rubber, others are virtually tasteless. If you are going to use condoms for oral sex, you might prefer to use one that is unlubricated.

Some are more messy to use than others. Condoms which are lubricated with silicone-based products tend to be less sticky and the lubricant is more evenly spread. A few brands are lubricated with the spermicide nonoxynol-9. Some women are allergic to this and find it irritates their skin. If you do get an allergic reaction using a condom for any kind of sex, try switching to a different brand, such as Durex Fetherlite, or use condoms which don't have any spermicidal lubrication. (If it is the rubber rather than the lubricant that you are sensitive to, try a condom like Durex Allergy.)

The colour and shape of the condom is your choice! Some condoms have a teat or reservoir at the tip, others are plain-ended. If you prefer

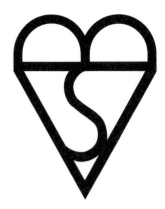

British Standard Institute Kitemark

> **Condoms**
> Apart from safety, you might want to consider:
> their taste and smell
> ease of opening the packet
> how easy they are to put on
> how they feel during sex
> whether they cause an irritation
> appearance
> texture
> cost

HOW TO USE

Always use a new condom. Check the expiry date on the pack before use.

Take the condom out of the package carefully. *Do not unroll it.* You'll never get it on that way! Be careful not to damage the rubber with fingernails or jewellery.

Many men produce some secretion from the penis (pre-cum) prior to ejaculation. To avoid any risk from pre-cum put the condom on after the penis has become hard but before you have genital contact.

With your thumb and forefinger, gently squeeze the tip of the condom at the closed end to expel the air. Air-bubbles can cause condoms to break. If the condom has no teat, make sure that you leave about half an inch free at the tip to catch the semen. Squeezing a dab of water-based lubricant inside the tip of the condom will help keep air out.

Hold the condom at the tip of the penis and with your other hand unroll it down to the base of the penis. If the man is uncircumcised pull back his foreskin before rolling on the condom. If the condom does not reach to the base of the penis, your partner should not penetrate beyond the condom base as this can cause the condom to come off inside you.

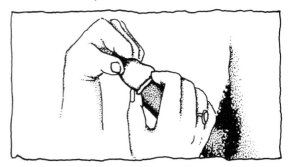

CONDOMS

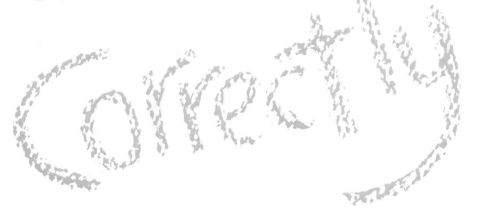

Make sure that the vagina or anus and the outside of the condom are well lubricated with a water-based lubricant before intercourse. Insufficient lubrication may cause condoms to tear or come off. Do not use oil-based lubricants as they damage the rubber.

Sometimes, for example if the penis is getting soft, the condom may tend to slip and certain sexual positions, for example when a woman is sitting on top of a man, can also cause the condom to come off. If the condom begins to slip, holding onto the base will help it stay put. This also feels nice for your partner and means that you can stimulate yourself too.

After intercourse, the man should withdraw before his penis gets soft. As he withdraws he should hold the condom around the base to avoid spilling the contents or losing the condom inside the vagina or anus.

Throw the used condom away! If you wrap it in a tissue it should flush down the toilet quite easily.

Condoms should not be used more than once – use a new condom *every* time you have intercourse.

this type make sure you leave a space at the end for the semen so that it doesn't get forced up the sides or cause the condom to break. Ribbed condoms have little bumps on the outside which are supposed to provide extra sensation for the woman; some women like them, but others find them irritating.

Most condoms are made of rubber but you can get condoms made from natural sheep-gut membranes. These are more expensive and are not recommended for safer sex. Homemade condoms made from cling film, crisp packets or saran wrap are definitely *not* safe either!

Several new brands of condoms have appeared recently which aim to reduce the risk and the worry associated with the condom breaking or slipping off. Mentor condoms, for example, have an adhesive on the inside of the rubber that sticks to the penis so that the condom won't slip off even if the penis becomes soft, or if you are on top. After making love it can be gently peeled off. Mentor also comes with an applicator which simplifies putting the condom on and makes it virtually impossible to unroll the condom the wrong way. The big disadvantage is that Mentor condoms are made in the United States and are not, at present, easily available in the UK – but this may change. They are also about 3 times as expensive as most other condoms.

Another recent development is a condom for women called Femshield. This is inserted into the vagina and once in place it fits over a woman's vulva. The good thing about a condom for women is that instead of having to rely on a man's co-operation, you can decide to protect yourself. On the other hand you could ask who this new condom has been developed for and why only now? Is it so men who don't want to be bothered using condoms can continue to leave responsibility for safer sex up to women? Another disadvantage is that some women who have tested the condom say it dulls sensation for them. Femshield is not yet available many countries.

Condoms make sex safer; they can also make sex more fun – watching your partner put on a condom or putting it on him can be exciting. You might like to experiment with different ways of putting them on or have fun trying out condoms in different colours (if it's Monday it must be purple!). Think of other ways you might play with condoms: stretch them over your mouth and see what it's like to kiss your partner; blow one up and tie a knot in the end; brush it across your partner's body, over their nipples, thighs, stomach and genitals, or use it to stimulate your labia and clitoris while masturbating or making love. (Don't insert it inside your vagina in case it bursts, and don't use condoms that have been stretched or blown up for intercourse.) Try squeezing or sucking it as if it were a breast or a penis. Get your partner to use their mouth to unroll a condom over your fingers and then feel their body through the rubber. When you masturbate fantasize about sex with condoms. Try putting a condom on your fingers and stimulating yourself. The more you and your partner associate condoms with sex you both find enjoyable, the more you will find using them arousing.

Some men, who have a tendency to come very quickly, find that by wearing a condom they can help delay ejaculation, giving both them and their partner more satisfaction. For men who have problems maintaining an erection, wearing a condom which fits tightly will tend to make erections harder and orgasms more intense. Condoms, especially the lubricated variety, also reduce friction and this can help to make intercourse a more pleasurable experience for women, especially if they are dry. Many women and men also find that because they are less worried about the various health risks associated with intercourse when they use condoms they are more able to relax and enjoy making love.

Condom-fun

SPERMICIDES AND LUBRICANTS

SPERMICIDAL LUBRICANTS

CREAMS AND JELLIES	WATER SOLUBLE/ WATER-BASED	NONOXYNOL-9
Delfen Cream	√	5%
Duracreme	√	*
Gynol II	√	2%
Ortho-Creme	√	2%
Staycept	√	6%

FOAMS		
Delfen Foam	√	12.5%

PESSARIES		
Orthoforms	√	5%
Two's Company	√	5%

FILM		
C-Film	√	67 mm

LUBRICANTS

KY Jelly	√	–
Duragel	√	*
Probe	√	–
Ortho Lubricant	√	–
Boots	√	–

* Both products contain Nonoxynol-11. Although studies have been carried out on Nonoxynol-9, it is likely that Nonoxynol-10 and 11 will also be effective against HIV.

Spermicides come in many varieties, including foams, gels, film, creams and pessaries. You can buy them over the counter at most chemists, by mail order or you can get them free from family planning clinics. All spermicides must be put in correctly if they are to help prevent pregnancy. The foams come with a plastic applicator that you use to insert the foam into your vagina (see photograph on page 39). It must be placed well inside so that the foam completely covers the cervix. Spermicidal pessaries must always be removed from their wrapper and, using your fingers, inserted high up in the vagina. After about 10 minutes the pessary should dissolve. (Check that the pessaries are not oil-based and liable to damage condoms.) Jellies and creams come in a tube with an applicator that you can use to insert the spermicide into your vagina.

Spermicides may not work if you use them incorrectly or if they have passed their expiry date. You should check the manufacturers' instructions on when you need to insert the spermicide before intercourse and how long you need to leave it in afterwards. It's possible for sperm to live in the vagina for several hours and so most spermicides should remain in for about 6 hours after intercourse. During this time you should not douche or have a bath as this can dilute or wash away the spermicide. You can still continue making love but remember that if you have intercourse again you will need to insert a further application of spermicidal jelly, cream, film or foam.

The contraceptive sponge contains the spermicide nonoxynol-9 and has the advantage that it remains effective for 24 hours, without any need for the reapplication of spermicide, so it provides protection regardless of how many times you have intercourse. Since it can be inserted either hours before intercourse or at the last moment, it is convenient as well. Many couples who have tried it also say that it doesn't stop their enjoyment of oral sex unlike many spermicidal products, which have an unpleasant taste. (Some women find that foams are better than jellies and cream for oral sex, but this is largely a matter for personal choice.) In addition to being tasteless and odourless, the sponge isn't as messy or drippy as some spermicidal products, but it is not an effective method of contraception on its own.

You can buy the contraceptive sponge, without a prescription, as with other spermicidal products, from most chemists. As with other products, to be effective it must be inserted properly and left in for at least 6 hours after intercourse. Before putting the sponge into your vagina you will need to wet it with a small amount of water until it feels moist and soapy but not dripping wet. This activates the spermicide in the sponge. It is then easily inserted by sliding it into the vagina as far as your fingers will go – rather like putting in a tampon. Check that the sponge is properly positioned and is covering your cervix by sliding your finger around the edge. Also, be sure that the string loop, which you pull to remove the sponge, dangles downwards.

The use of a spermicide or a lubricant may require you to stop what you are doing in order to apply it, but this doesn't have to be a passion-killer. You can make it a part of lovemaking. Of course it could rather spoil the mood if you have to spend ages rummaging in a drawer for a tube of spermicide or lubricant insisting, 'I know it's here somewhere!' Your partner could be asleep or half way to Timbuctoo by the time you find it. Be prepared – put spermicides and lubricants within easy reach, so that you don't have to get up and look for them.

If used correctly and consistently, spermicides can help to make sex safer. When used with another method of birth control, such as a diaphragm or condom, they reduce the risk of unplanned pregnancy. Spermicides also provide some protection from sexually transmitted diseases, such as gonorrhoea and herpes, and they may also give extra protection against the HIV virus, but only if they contain nonoxynol-9. This is a substance which has been used for years in contraceptive foams and gels because it kills sperm. But it has recently been found that, at least in the laboratory, it also kills the HIV virus. This does *not* mean that if you use a spermicide or a lubricant containing nonoxynol-9 you won't become infected with HIV because although it might work in a test-tube, we simply don't know how effective it is against the virus during intercourse. It goes without saying that a woman's vagina and a laboratory are very different environments. For this reason, spermicides and lubricants containing nonoxynol-9 should only be used as a backup to condoms, not by themselves.

If I use a spermicide or a lubricant with nonoxynol-9 in it, does that mean I don't need to bother using condoms?
Absolutely not! Condoms by themselves offer very good protection against HIV and other sexually transmitted diseases. Using nonoxynol-9 is like adding another layer of protection in case the condom should break or fall off. Nonoxynol-9 without a condom does not provide adequate protection against infection or pregnancy.

It should say on the packet whether a spermicide or lubricant contains nonoxynol-9, if it doesn't, consult the guide to spermicides and lubricants on page 128 or ask at the chemist. Most spermicides, at present, contain between 1% and 5% of nonoxynol-9; foams contain the highest concentration – up to 12%.

What to look out for

How effective a product is will depend on how good it is at providing a physical as well as a chemical barrier against sperm and viruses. As well as containing more nonoxynol-9, foams are very good at forming a thick barrier that sperm can't swim through. They also spread more evenly and cling to the walls of the vagina better than other types of spermicides – gels are the worst.

A few women and men are allergic to nonoxynol-9 and may find certain spermicidal products make them sore. If nonoxynol-9 or any other spermicidal ingredient irritates your vagina, it could make it easier for the HIV virus to enter the bloodstream. Test any product containing nonoxynol-9 on the side of your

131

wrist first before using it for sex or try it out vaginally on your own. If you do get an allergic reaction try a different brand.

Nonoxynol-9 has been approved for use during vaginal intercourse and oral sex. What isn't clear is whether it can be safely used during anal sex. The concern is that it may irritate the delicate walls of the rectum, creating a possible route for infection. (The lining on the inside of the mouth and vagina is much thicker and tougher than that of the anus.) You might try using lubricants on your own to see if you become irritated or sore.

Lubricants

Lubrication is an important part of safer sex. Apart from helping to prevent condoms from breaking or being pulled off, the use of a lubricant during vaginal and anal intercourse will help to reduce friction and possible injury to the walls of the vagina or rectum, which might allow the HIV virus or other infections to enter your bloodstream. Lubrication also makes penetration and clitoral stimulation more pleasurable. Saliva is a good natural lubricant (it's easier to lick your fingers than reach for a tube) but its ability to reduce friction is short-lived, making tissue injury more likely. If you make love with a woman and use your lubrication to wet her, or she does this to you, there could be a risk of passing on HIV and certain vaginal infections such as thrush and herpes (see pages 55 and 59).

•

I find that if I'm dry I don't enjoy being touched. Using a lubricant helps.

•

When I first used a lubricant I didn't much like it; it was too sticky. Now I've found one that feels more natural.

•

Choosing a lubricant

There are many different lubricants to choose from but as far as safer sex is concerned the best are ones that contain nonoxynol-9 and are water-based, like KY or Duragel. Oil-based lubricants like baby oil, Vaseline, margarine, hand creams or massage oils should not be used because they rot the rubber which condoms, diaphragms and latex barriers are made of. This doesn't mean that if you use oil on a condom it will suddenly fall apart but it will get thinner and tend to break more easily. Also, oil-based lubricants tend to trap germs and, because they are harder to clean off, they tend to linger longer.

•

I love the slippery feel it gives.

•

I find using a lubricant increases sensation – but not if it's cold. Keep it in a warm place!

•

It's important to use *water-based* lubricants with condoms or latex barriers, not those that are merely *water-soluble*. The water-soluble lubricants may wash out of your sheets but they still contain oil. Spermicidal products may give extra lubrication as well as providing some protection against infection and pregnancy but again make sure that they are not oil-based. It should say on the packet whether a lubricant or spermicide is water or oil-based and if it contains nonoxynol-9. Check the lubricant chart on page 128.

Water-based versus water-soluble

You can buy lubricants like KY jelly from any chemist and from companies that sell condoms and other 'sex-aids' by mail order. Try out different brands and see which you like best. Apart from safety, the kind of things that may affect your choice are:

What to think about

• The smell and taste.   Some lubricants have virtually no smell or taste, others may have rather a sharp, chemical taste or may be slightly sweet.

• How long do they last?   Some lubricants dry out quicker than others, but many water-based lubricants have a second life and become slippery again if you wet them.

• How well do they lubricate?   This depends on what you intend to use them for. A lubricant which is gummy and dries out fairly quickly isn't going to be very good for penetrative sex, either from the point of view of safety or pleasure.

• Texture.   Some products are transparent, slippery and runny; others are gooey or sticky and feel less natural.

• How do they feel on your body?   Do you like the sensation of some lubricants more than others? Which are the most fun to use in massaging and touching your partner's body?

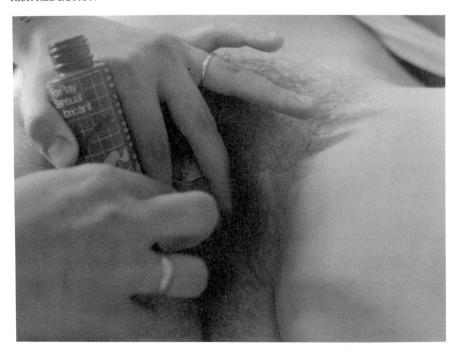

Apart from the safer sex benefits, the use of a lubricant can improve the enjoyment you get out of sex if you are dry. A small dab of water-based lubricant in the tip of a condom can increase sensation for a man, as well as helping to keep air out and so prevent the condom breaking. And you can also have fun in other ways. Use them for massaging your partner's body or instead rub on a flavoured kind and enjoy kissing and licking it off.

CHAPTER FIVE

NEGOTIATING

SAFER

SEX

If you have read this book from start to finish, you will know a great deal about safer sex by now; what it is and what it can protect you from. This will be of no use, however, unless you can negotiate ways of making love safely with your partner and so this chapter looks at some of the ways we can start to put what we know about safer sex into practice.

For some of us this is not going to be a problem. We can be assertive: we can suggest changes in lovemaking, say we don't want to have certain kinds of sex, buy condoms, dental dams and lubricants. On the other hand, it's also true to say that many of us don't find it that easy to negotiate safer sex. Let's begin by looking at some of the reasons for this.

Many of us have great difficulty talking about sex with our partners, sometimes this is because we feel too embarrassed and shy or perhaps we don't feel it's quite right for us to tell our partner what we'd like them to do. Often it's because we don't know what words to use – we don't have a language for talking about sex that's easy to use. Words like intercourse or vagina may feel too medical and formal and other expressions, like 'foreplay' or 'make love', are too vague to communicate very much. This leaves words like fuck, screw, cunt,

How to say you want safer sex

●

It's sometimes hard to know what to say.

●

135

tits, cock which, because they are often used as insults, we may find too offensive or crude.

Whether we use medical terms, slang or euphemistic expressions like 'let's go to bed', the language of sex reflects and reinforces the idea that sex equals penetration. How many words or expressions can you think of to mean intercourse? What about other, safer ways of making love such as 'mutual masturbation', body rubbing, kissing and cunnilingus: can you come up with as many words to describe these? The vocabulary of sex is much more concerned with describing what happens to a man's body during sexual arousal.

Other problems can arise if you or your partner talk about sex in a way the other doesn't like. Negotiating safer sex is not just about communicating what you want to do together, it's also about agreeing on how to describe what you want. If your partner uses words that you find offensive or unacceptable, you are not going to feel like making love very much. One way of agreeing on language you both find acceptable is to say, or write down, some of the words for different sexual activities and parts of the body. Which do you both feel comfortable using? You could turn to the Glossary on page 154 and point to words you feel OK about and those you don't.

If you do not like using certain words or if you can't think of any that would describe what it is you are feeling or thinking, you could make up your own expressions; ones that you feel safe about and you enjoy. I know a couple who have developed a code for different positions: apple turnover and cupcake! This may not be a language which turns you on, but you can always develop your own sexual vocabulary to use with your partner.

If you don't talk about sex you may end up making love in ways that are not only unsafe but also not very enjoyable. When you have trouble finding words to express what you want to do, you can always *show* your partner exactly what you really like. This is easier for some people than telling someone in words and it can be a lot of fun! It also leaves fewer doubts about what someone means when they say, 'I'd like you to touch me more firmly' or 'I'd love it if you moved your hand a little to the left.' You might hold your partner's hand and guide them to where you would like to be touched; let them feel the kind of movement you prefer.

Sometimes the problem is letting your partner know the kinds of sex you enjoy and feel safe doing. This might mean talking about using a condom or having non-penetrative sex. Suggestions for how you might do this are discussed later, on page 144.

An important aspect of safer sex is being able to be assertive in sexual relationships. It's no good having a language to talk about sex with if you don't feel able to say what you want. Words are useless if you don't feel able to introduce the topic.

You may be someone who feels confident enough to do this but many women are lacking in confidence when it comes to sex. Sometimes this is because they feel that to be sexually assertive would lead to problems or that it is not something that they think that they have a right to be. One of the reasons why women experience sex this way is that we are brought up to regard our own pleasure as less important than someone else's. Traditionally women are often expected to play a passive role, in which the man takes the initative and the woman is expected to satisfy his needs regardless of whether this is what she wants and enjoys. However much we may disagree, it can be difficult to ignore such pressures. This is why we often feel guilty or demanding if we talk about sex and what gives *us* pleasure.

The first step in learning to be more assertive in sexual relationships is recognising that you have a right to say how you feel and how *you* would like to make love. Be honest about your feelings. Your partner may not necessarily like what you have to say but no one can dispute the way you feel. You are the person who knows about what you like and feel, and if your partner is to relate to you, rather than a false image of how they would like you to be,

Sexual confidence

•

I sometimes feel I don't have the right to ask.

•

Some people think that women shouldn't talk about sex.

•

137

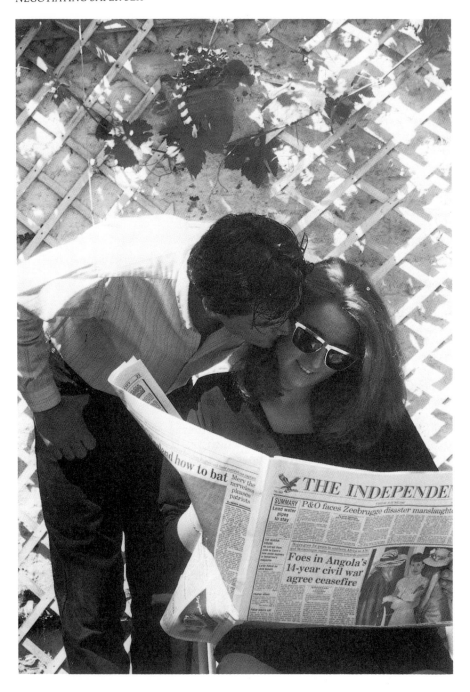

it's important that they acknowledge how you are feeling. Another aspect of stressing your feelings is that it might help to avoid feelings of hurt and rejection or anger in a partner. It's not that you are saying that what they do is necessarily wrong, it's just that it's not what *you* want.

The next stage is to make an agreement with yourself that you will only have sex if it is *your* kind of safer sex. Once you are clear in your own mind about what you want, it will be easier to talk about it with others and you will be less likely to be talked out of it. Even then, you may find that you have to be very determined and repeat things several times before your partner will acknowledge how you are feeling and what you want.

You are probably going to be more successful if you express your needs in a positive way. For example, instead of saying 'You don't touch me the way I want you to', you might say something like 'I love it when we are making love and you stroke my breasts'. Or you might take their hand and show them. This way you are suggesting changes rather than just criticising what your partner does. It's also important to choose a time to talk about safer sex when you can both discuss how you feel (see page 143).

Once you've raised the subject of safer sex the next stage is to negotiate what you can do together. You might ask 'What's your idea of safer sex?' or if you are embarrassed it might be easier, as well as a lot of fun, to make a game out of finding out. This can be a time to explore, play and become intimate with another person.

Write down five safer sex activities that you would like to try, putting each one on a separate piece of paper. Get your partner to do the same, then fold the pieces of paper in two. Take it in turns to select one and then read out what it says or, if you quite like the idea, get your partner to guess which of their suggestions you have chosen by trying it out! Another version of this is for you both to make a list of some of the things you like doing in bed – or wherever you enjoy making love. Then each make a list of the things you wouldn't feel safe doing and swop lists. Are there some things that are on both lists? Are there parts of your lists that are easier to negotiate than others? Alternatively, you could always lend your partner a copy of this book to read, with the things you'd like to do helpfully underlined in green for go!

Don't expect too much of yourself too soon. Learning to be assertive in sex isn't going to happen overnight. It's something that develops gradually out of your experience of coping with different situations. And if you feel you want to learn more about becoming assertive you could think about going on an assertion training course or getting a book to help. Check with local libraries, colleges or women's groups to see what's available.

What will my partner think?

Another reason why we don't always find it easy to say what we feel is that we are concerned about how our partner will react – they might be hurt or they might become annoyed, even violent. We might worry about being rejected or that they will leave. We may also be worried about how talking about safer sex makes us look.

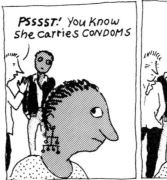 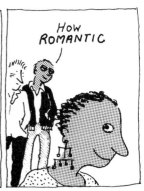

●

If you carry condoms men think you're on the lookout for sex.

●

Many women feel that raising the subject of safer sex, especially using a condom, is to risk being seen as an 'easy-lay' – being prepared means that you are asking for it, and your sexual knowledge shows that you've been around. This is the old sexual double-standard at work. We don't talk about men being slags or

140

tarts if they say they want or enjoy sex – men gain status through having sex – but if women do this they still risk getting a bad reputation.

Double standards like this can make it very difficult for women to put what they know about safer sex into practice. Men often *assume* that a woman is on the pill or using some other method of contraception – it's women who get pregnant so it's their business! Similarly, although both women and men get AIDS and other sexually transmitted diseases, like herpes and gonorrhoea, men can often be just as lax about protecting themselves and their partners from disease. It is usually assumed that women take this on. Responsibility for the safety of sex should be shared, yet the catch is that when women are prepared with condoms, or suggest ways of making love that don't involve inter-course, they sometimes find that men don't respect them, or that they react defensively by refusing to discuss it or getting angry. The expectation is that men should take the sexual initiative rather than women.

This is one reason why some men may resist talking about safer sex. Another is the threat this poses to their identity and self-esteem.

Not all men will feel upset or insulted if you talk to them about safer sex; they may have been thinking of ways to introduce the subject them-selves and feel relieved that you've mentioned it. Other men are threatened if their sexual power is challenged in this way. In our society having sex, especially intercourse, is very closely linked with being masculine for men; it can be a way of proving oneself, of gaining status and power and, consequently, it can be an area of vulnerability. (This is not to say that women don't feel vulnerable in their sexuality; but a woman's self-esteem is more likely to be associated with being sexually attractive than with her sexual 'performance'.) That's why some women are reluctant to suggest to a man ways they would like lovemaking to change; they may feel that this will put them more at risk, not less.

●

You can't win; if you carry condoms you're fast, if you don't you're blamed for being irresponsible.

●

Men's attitudes towards sex

141

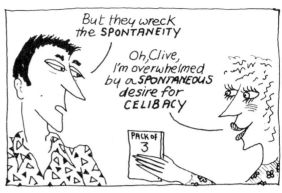

Not wanting to upset your partner, especially if you are afraid, is understandable enough and it's difficult to make changes if you are socially and economically dependent on someone. But remember when we don't say what we want in order to keep someone else happy, it's our health, our sexual pleasure, our self-esteem and our relationship, that we are putting at risk.

A man might also presume that safer sex is not erotic and assume he won't enjoy it. While some men realise that safer sex can be both satisfying and fun, to many good sex means not wearing a condom when they have intercourse. To them safer sex may seem dull and boring, a poor substitute for the 'real-thing'. They have a lot to learn about sex! As we discussed earlier in the book, there are lots of pleasurable ways to make love. With partners who are reluctant to change you might point out that to define sex only as penetration is very limiting. Don't they at least want to know what they are missing out on?

Often when someone says that they can't change, what they really mean is: I don't want to change. While it may not be easy for a person to change their sexual habits, it clearly is possible to develop new ways of relating to other people sexually. (For many of us this is part of the fun of having sex with someone.) Many gay men, for instance, have changed their sexual practices in the light of AIDS.

Next time your partner says that they can't change, get them to explain what they mean.

Maybe they feel there's no reason to change, that safer sex is only for people who are gay, inject drugs or sleep around. If this is the case they need to become more sex-wise!

Power and control

The degree of control women have within a relationship will seriously affect whether they feel able to talk to their partners about what they can do together. Some women have control over some situations but not others – again, it can be easier to be assertive with someone you've just begun a relationship with than with someone on whom you are economically and emotionally dependent. Other women may be financially independent from their partner but still feel they lack control in the relationship because they are frightened of being left alone and all that that means. Sex can't be seen in isolation from the rest of our lives. Because women are rarely accorded the same privileges, status and power as men, they are often not in a position to insist on condoms or making love without having intercourse. To do so might be difficult and also dangerous.

These sorts of problems can't be solved by reading a book, or going on an assertiveness training course. The difficulties some women experience in negotiating safer sex only serve to highlight wider social problems for women. New job opportunities, equal pay, day care facilities, affordable housing for women living alone, battered women's refuges, are just some of the things that some women need to be safe in their relationships.

There are a number of organisations listed on page 161 which offer help to women in violent or abusive relationships.

Choose the right time

If possible, you should try to talk with your partner about what you can do together *before* you start making love. When you are aroused, kissing and caressing each other, is not the best moment for a discussion. Pick a moment when your head can rule your heart and you're not worried about spoiling the mood. It is tempting to have a few drinks to help you pluck up the courage to discuss safer sex but alcohol can

143

impair your judgement, and you may end up saying and doing things that you later regret. It's also a good idea to avoid using drugs as a way of making you feel more relaxed about talking these things over.

Choose a time when you are able to talk without being interrupted and when you both feel relaxed. Don't wait until you've just had a row, a really dreadful day at work, when you are feeling tired and sleepy, just before you are about to have visitors or on your way out. This is likely to produce a different kind of response to discussing the whole issue while you are having a cosy evening together, or a relaxing weekend away from it all.

After you've given some thought to when you might raise the subject of safer sex, the next question is *how*?

How to talk about safer sex

Some couples find it easy to talk to each other about their relationship, including sex. Others have to work at learning how to communicate with each other. This is part of the agony and the ecstasy of getting to know someone, but where should you start?

One way to begin a conversation about safer sex, especially with someone you don't know very well, is to talk about AIDS generally. It probably isn't a good idea to start with 'Would you like to know the figures on how many people have got AIDS through sex?' but you might mention a television programme or newspaper article which discussed AIDS. Given the anxieties many of us have about talking about sex this is often considerably easier than launching straight into a discussion of what the pair of you can do safely together. It can also give you some insight into what this person is really like and, in particular, how open they are to discussing the need for safer sex and all that this implies.

If this approach doesn't lead to a discussion about your relationship, then you may need to try a more direct approach – the 'I really like you but before we get any more involved I need to talk to you about something' approach. And it might go on like this:

There's a lot of talk these days about AIDS, does that ever worry you?

Hang on a minute, are you saying I've got AIDS?

No, but AIDS has made me think about the way I make love. Hasn't it you?

What are you trying to tell me?

I want to have sex with you but if we do we should both protect ourselves and have safer sex.

You don't need to worry about that stuff with me.

Like I said, I really want to have sex with you, but if we do I want us to have safer sex.

What do you mean, safer sex?

Well, lots of things. We could use a condom for a start or . . . Come on! This could be a lot of fun.

You must be joking!

Why not try? You never know you might really enjoy yourself!

No way!

Don't you want to make love?

Yes, but not with a condom.

Acknowledging that this is an awkward or embarrassing topic for you, if it is, may help take some of the pressure off. If you don't find it easy, say so! You may, on the other hand, prefer to get straight to the point by saying something simple and straightforward like 'Have you used a condom?' or 'What brand of condoms have you tried?'

If you can agree on some safer sex alternatives, that's great! If not, the conversation might end something like this:

You know that I want to make love with you, but if we don't have safer sex then you can forget it! I won't do it unsafely.

Every relationship is different and consequently what works with one person won't

145

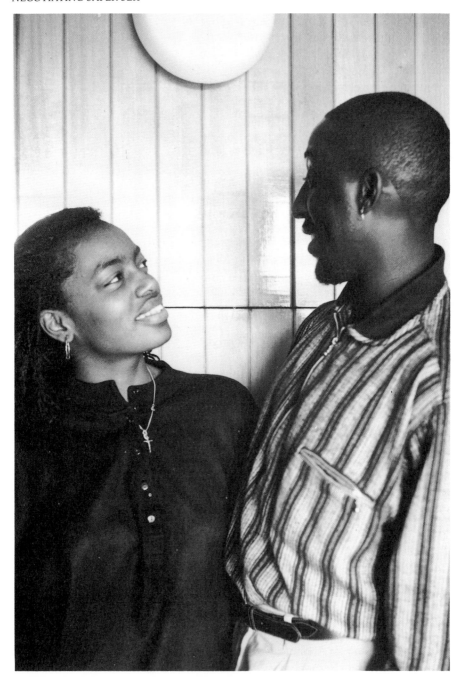

work with another. How you deal with the situation will also depend on whether you've just met or not. It may be easier to say what you want to a new partner because nothing is established yet. But it can also be more difficult talking about sex with someone you don't know very well.

You'll have to decide on your own approach. Whatever you decide to say, you need to be prepared for your partner's reaction. They may appreciate what you say and respect your honesty and courage in bringing up a subject that most people find hard to talk about. It is also possible that they will react negatively.

Is your partner willing to play safe? If initially they become angry or annoyed because you want to discuss safer sex tell them how you feel. Emphasize your own feelings so that you do not seem to be accusing or criticising (instead of 'you never . . .', try 'I really like it when' or 'I feel . . .' rather than 'you're making me feel').

If they give you a hard time by trying to make you feel guilty, by saying 'Don't you trust me?' or 'If you really loved me, you'd do it without a condom', stick to your guns. Don't give way to emotional blackmail. Look them in the eye and tell them that wanting to have safer sex has nothing to do with not liking them or not finding them attractive. It's not meant as an insult and you are not just talking about protecting yourself. Safer sex means protecting each other.

Similarly, don't be pressurized into having sex because he says he won't love you any more if you don't or that he will love you forever if you do. This can be hard but your health, your self-esteem and your relationship may depend on learning to stand up for yourself.

One way of tackling the condom question, is to act as if you expect him to use one: 'I can hardly wait to get the condoms out' or 'Can you believe that in this day and age that some men expect to go to bed with someone without bothering to use a condom!' This might work, especially if he doesn't want to seem old-fashioned! If he claims not to have used condoms

Anticipating difficulties

before tell him you'll be happy to help him practice. If he says he wouldn't mind using one but doesn't have any with him, take one out. If he asks you what kind of a woman you are carrying condoms, tell him you are a woman who wants to live a long and healthy life and you expect he does too.

If anyone accuses you of being a kill-joy and spoiling the mood, you could say you're sorry for choosing the wrong moment but there will be other times to feel like that again. If they say 'What's the matter with you, don't you like sex?' or 'Are you hung up, going off sex or something?' then make it clear that that's not what you are saying and that you do like sex and want to make love (if that's the case). Offer some suggestions about the things you might do. Safer sex is great sex, there's no need to feel apologetic about it. Emphasize that you can have a lot of fun putting a condom on, or making love in ways they may not have tried before. They might be persuaded! But if you don't feel you can trust somebody not to try to force you to have unprotected intercourse, then it's safer not to get into a situation where this may happen.

Your partner may refuse to take no for an answer and insist on having sex the way they want it, however risky. If this is the case you must seriously ask yourself if you want a relationship with someone who doesn't respect your wishes, and is willing to put both themselves and you at risk. Ultimately, only you can decide whether what you get from your relationship is worth the risk, but it may help to talk it through with friends or with someone at one of the organisations listed on page 161.

Ending a relationship is more difficult in some situations than others. For some women it is unrealistic and not what they really want to happen. One way of suggesting changes in lovemaking in a long-standing relationship is to use general health concerns. This is also a useful strategy in situations where your partner is likely to interpret your desire to practise safer sex to mean that you have been seeing someone else.

UNREASONABLE DEMANDS

Here are a few examples of below-the-belt comments to watch out for:

You don't want to have intercourse! Well why did you say you wanted to make love in the first place then?
This man has a lot to learn, can you wait that long?

So you think I'm gay do you?
Safer sex is something we all need to think about, it's not just about gay men.

Safer sex is boring.
Any sex is boring if the people doing it are boring – sounds as though this person has limited imagination.

Don't worry, I've had a vasectomy.
Safer sex isn't just about not getting pregnant – it's about protecting *both* of you from infections that you may not even know you have.

You say you don't want to do this, but I know you really want to.
Is he listening to what you're saying? When you say no you mean no!

You're making me lose my erection.
That's OK, you've got plenty of time!

What, do you think I have a disease or something?
No, you're not saying that. It's just that if you have intercourse you make it a rule for yourself to always use a condom.

Feelings must be acknowledged if they are to be dealt with and you shouldn't ignore the way your partner feels, just as they can't deny the way you feel. But this *doesn't mean* that you should go along with what they want because they are feeling rejected or upset. However much you may care about a person, if you say yes to what they want when it's not what you want, you run the risk of eventually hating and resenting both of you. Sex where you say yes when you mean no is not safe. It can seriously affect you, as well as possibly putting you at risk of an unplanned pregnancy or of becoming infected with HIV or sexually transmitted diseases.

Safer sex is an opportunity to consider your relationships in a different light. Being able to discuss with your partner what you want to do can improve the quality of your relationship generally, it can also improve your sex-life. It may even save your life.

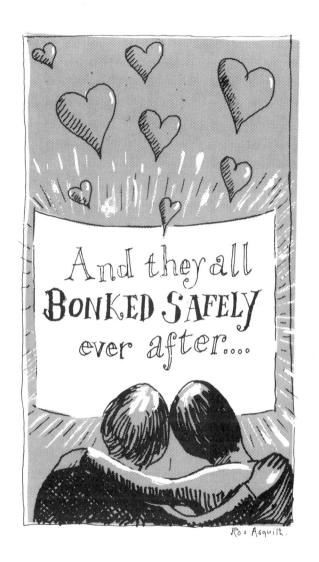

MENSTRUAL CALENDAR

Circle the date when your period starts.

A horizontal line indicates a regular 28 day cycle.

A line sloping down from left to right indicates a longer cycle (28 days plus the number of days below the level of your last period).

A line sloping upwards indicates a shorter cycle (28 days plus the number of days above the level of your last period).

If there is no straight line, your period is irregular.

JAN	JAN FEB	FEB MAR	MAR APR	APR MAY	MAY JUN	JUN JUL	JUL AUG	AUG SEP	SEP OCT	OCT NOV	NOV DEC	DEC	DEC JAN
1	29	26	26	23	21	18	16	13	10	8	5	3	31
2	30	27	27	24	22	19	17	14	11	9	6	4	JAN 1
3	31	28	28	25	23	20	18	15	12	10	7	5	2
4	FEB 1	MAR 1	29	26	24	21	19	16	13	11	8	6	3
5	2	2	30	27	25	22	20	17	14	12	9	7	4
6	3	3	31	28	26	23	21	18	15	13	10	8	5
7	4	4	APR 1	29	27	24	22	19	16	14	11	9	6
8	5	5	2	30	28	25	23	20	17	15	12	10	7
9	6	6	3	MAY 1	29	26	24	21	18	16	13	11	8
10	7	7	4	2	30	27	25	22	19	17	14	12	9
11	8	8	5	3	31	28	26	23	20	18	15	13	10
12	9	9	6	4	JUN 1	29	27	24	21	19	16	14	11
13	10	10	7	5	2	30	28	25	22	20	17	15	12
14	11	11	8	6	3	JUL 1	29	26	23	21	18	16	13
15	12	12	9	7	4	2	30	27	24	22	19	17	14
16	13	13	10	8	5	3	31	28	25	23	20	18	15
17	14	14	11	9	6	4	AUG 1	29	26	24	21	19	16
18	15	15	12	10	7	5	2	30	27	25	22	20	17
19	16	16	13	11	8	6	3	31	28	26	23	21	18
20	17	17	14	12	9	7	4	SEP 1	29	27	24	22	19
21	18	18	15	13	10	8	5	2	30	28	25	23	20
22	19	19	16	14	11	9	6	3	OCT 1	29	26	24	21
23	20	20	17	15	12	10	7	4	2	30	27	25	22
24	21	21	18	16	13	11	8	5	3	31	28	26	23
25	22	22	19	17	14	12	9	6	4	NOV 1	29	27	24
26	23	23	20	18	15	13	10	7	5	2	30	28	25
27	24	24	21	19	16	14	11	8	6	3	DEC 1	29	26
28	25	25	22	20	17	15	12	9	7	4	2	30	27

153

GLOSSARY

AIDS Acquired Immune Deficiency Syndrome is believed to be caused by the HIV virus which breaks down the body's immune system. As a result, people who have AIDS become susceptible to certain opportunistic infections and cancers.

Anal intercourse (back or rear entry, buggery, Greek, sodomy, arse-fucking) This is a form of sexual intercourse where a man puts his penis inside the anus of a woman or a man.

Analingus (rimming, reaming) Licking, kissing, sucking someone's anus.

Antibodies Protein molecules produced by the body in response to an infection. The antibodies produced to fight infection with HIV are not usually effective.

Antibody positive A blood test result showing that a person has been infected with the HIV virus and has developed antibodies to it. It does *not* mean that a person has AIDS.

Anus (arsehole, bum-hole) The opening at the lower end of the bowel.

Areola The circle of dark skin around the nipple.

Bisexual (AC/DC) A person who is sexually attracted to both men and women.

Celibacy Abstaining from sex. Some people include masturbation under their definition of celibacy, others do not.

Cervical cap A small plastic or rubber contraceptive device which fits over the cervix to provide a barrier against sperm.

154

Cervix The neck of the uterus which protrudes into the vagina.

Chlamydia A vaginal or urinary infection which can be sexually transmitted.

Clitoris A small, complex organ situated where the inside lips of the vagina meet; its only known function is erotic pleasure. It plays a crucial role in a woman's orgasm.

Condom (French letter, sheath, rubber, johnny) A thin rubber sheath worn over a man's penis to prevent pregnancy, sexually transmitted diseases and infection with HIV.

Cunnilingus (eat, French, go down on, licking out, oral sex) When a person uses their mouth to lick, kiss, suck a woman's genitals.

Diaphragm A dome-shaped rubber contraceptive device inserted into the vagina to cover the cervix; it must be used with a spermicide to be effective.

Douche Using a liquid to rinse the vagina or rectum.

Ejaculation (come, cum, shoot your load) Emission of semen from the penis.

Erection (hard on) When a man's penis becomes hard.

Faeces (waste products, excrement, shit) Scat is a slang term for sexual activities that involve faeces.

Fellatio (cock-sucking, blow-job, French, giving head, go down on, oral sex) When someone uses their mouth and tongue to stimulate a man's penis.

Fisting (fist-fucking, handballing) This is the term used to describe someone inserting their hand into another person's vagina or rectum.

Frottage (body rubbing) Sexual excitement from rubbing against another person's (clothed) body.

Gay Someone who finds others of the same gender sexually attractive and defines themselves as such (see also Homosexual, Lesbian).

Genitalia (privates) In women this area is called the vulva and customarily refers to the inner and outer lips (labia) of the vagina and the clitoris. In men this term refers to the penis, testicles and scrotum.

Genito-urinary clinic (see STD clinic).

Gonorrhoea (clap, a dose) A sexually transmitted disease caused by bacteria. Untreated it can cause complications, especially infertility in women.

G spot	(Grafenberg spot) A region of the front wall of the vagina claimed to have a high degree of erotic sensitivity.
Herpes	Viral infection of herpes simplex 1 or 2, which produces painful blisters in the mouth, anus or genital area and is sexually transmitted.
Heterosexual	(straight) A term used to describe sexual relationships between women and men.
HIV	Human Immunodeficiency Virus; this is the name researchers have agreed upon for the virus which causes AIDS.
HIV Antibody Test	A blood test which shows whether or not a person has antibodies to the HIV virus.
Homosexual	(gay) Used to describe sex between two men and, sometimes, two women. Also used to describe a person who is homosexual or gay (see also Lesbian).
Hymen	(maidenhead) A thin tissue covering the opening of the vagina which is usually broken quite naturally without a girl even knowing.
Immune system	The bodily system which fights infection.
Intercourse	(fucking, screwing, penetration, having sex, making love) Sex where a man puts his penis into a woman's vagina is called vaginal intercourse. When he puts it into a man or woman's rectum (back-passage) this is called anal intercourse.
Intra-uterine device	(IUD) A small metal or plastic object inserted into the uterus to prevent pregnancy.
Labia	The lips of the vagina. Labia majora refers to the two outer folds of skin; labia minora refers to the inner lips enclosing the urethral and vaginal openings.
Lesbian	(dyke, lezzie, gay) A woman who finds other women sexually attractive and defines herself as such.
Massage	Caressing and stroking the body for sensual/sexual enjoyment or relaxation.
Mastectomy	Surgical removal of the breast.
Masturbation	(jacking off, fiddling, frigging, playing with yourself, wanking) Making yourself sexually excited by touching your own body.
Menstruation	(the curse, monthly blues, period, on the rag) The bleeding associated with the shedding of the lining of the uterus, which occurs about once a month in most women from puberty until their late forties or early fifties.

Monogamous	(being faithful) Having sex only with the person you are having a relationship with.
Mons pubis	(mons veneris, mound of Venus) The cushion of fatty tissue over the bone in women which is covered in pubic hair.
Mutual masturbation	(hand job) Using your hands to stimulate each other's genitals at the same time, or taking turns. Additionally you can both masturbate in the presence of each other.
Nonoxynol-9	A chemical agent in some spermicides and lubricants which kills both sperms and the HIV virus. It is also effective against a wide range of sexually transmitted diseases.
Opportunistic infections	Infections which take advantage of the opportunity offered by the body's weakened immune system to cause illness.
Oral sex	When a person uses their mouth and tongue to stimulate another person's genitals (see also Analingus, Cunnilingus, Fellatio, Sixty-nine).
Penis	(cock, dick, willie, prick, shaft) Male sex organ which houses the urethra that carries both semen and urine (pee) out of the body.
Rectum	(back passage) The lower part of the bowel, ending in the anus.
Rimming	(see Analingus).
Safer sex	Ways of having sex that reduce the risk of contracting HIV or other sexually transmitted diseases, pregnancy, and physical or emotional abuse.
Sado-masochism	(S/M) When erotic stimulation is obtained through giving or receiving physical or psychological pain and/or humiliation.
Scrotum	The thin loose sac of skin just below the penis that contains the testicles.
Semen	(cum) The fluid containing sperm ejaculated from a man's penis.
Sero-positive	A person who has a positive test result after the HIV antibody test, which means they have antibodies to HIV in their blood (see also Antibody positive).
Sixty-nine	(soixante-neuf) Term for mutual oral sex.
Special clinic	(see STD clinic).
Speculum	A device used to hold the walls of the vagina apart to allow an examination.
Spermicide	A chemical substance that kills sperm (see also Nonoxynol-9).

157

STDs	An abbreviation for sexually transmitted diseases (see also VD).
STD clinic	(genito-urinary clinic, special clinic, VD clinic) A clinic which specialises in dealing with sexually transmitted diseases.
Syphilis	A sexually transmitted disease, now relatively rare, that in its final stages can cause serious heart problems, brain damage and paralysis.
Testicles	(balls, nuts) Located in the scrotum underneath the penis, the testicles produce sperm.
Thrush	A common yeast infection which makes you feel very itchy inside your vagina.
Tribadism	Sex between two women involving rubbing their bodies together.
Trichomoniasis	An infection of the vagina caused by bacteria.
Urethra	The tube which conducts urine from the bladder out of the body in women and urine or semen in men.
Urine	(wee, piss, pee).
Uterus	(womb) A hollow, pear-shaped organ which is part of the female internal reproductive system, in which the fertilised egg becomes embedded and develops into a foetus during pregnancy. It is the lining of the uterus which is shed during a woman's period (see also Menstruation).
Vagina	(cunt) The organ in women leading from the vulva to the uterus.
Vaginal intercourse	(coitus, copulation, fucking, having sex, penetration, screwing) Sex where a man puts his penis in a woman's vagina.
Vaginitis	Vaginal inflammation from infection or chemical irritation.
Vasectomy	Sterilisation of a man by cutting and tying the tubes which carry sperm from the testes.
VD	Abbreviation for venereal disease. Infection spread through sexual intercourse (see also STDs).
Vulva	Term for external genitalia in women, the mons pubis, labia, clitoris and vaginal opening.
Watersports	(golden showers) Slang term for sexual activities that involve urine.
Withdrawal	(coitus interruptus) Removal of the penis from the vagina before ejaculation occurs.
Womb	(see Uterus).

FURTHER READING

The following books will give you further information on many of the issues raised in this book:

Meulenbelt, Anja, *For Ourselves* (Sheba, 1981)
Illustrated, it integrates personal experiences with information on sex, reproduction and sexual relationships with women and men. Clearly written in an easy to read style, but it doesn't cover AIDS, safer sex and prevention of sexually transmitted diseases.

Cousins-Mills, Jane, *Make it Happy, Make it Safe* (Penguin, 1988)
Written for young people, this easy to understand book contains lots of useful information about sex, AIDS, sexually transmitted diseases, contraception, abortion and pregnancy.

Phillips, Angela and Rakusen, Jill, *The New Our Bodies, Ourselves* (Penguin, 1989)
Still one of the best books which covers all aspects of women's health and sexuality. Updated edition of the 1978 classic.

Gordon, Peter and Mitchell, Louise, *Safer Sex* (Faber, 1988)
Written for both women and men this book is

helpful on suggestions for negotiating safer sex, but does not include detailed information on AIDS, sexually transmitted diseases, or birth control.

Kitzinger, Sheila, *Women's Experience of Sex* (Penguin, 1983)
Fully illustrated with photographs and drawings, this is a highly informative book on all aspects of sexuality, written in a style that incorporates women's personal experiences. It unfortunately does not discuss AIDS (or other sexually transmitted diseases) or how this has changed many people's expectations and experience of sex.

Richardson, Diane, *Women and the AIDS Crisis* (Pandora, 2nd ed, 1989)
Fully revised and up-dated edition of the first book to explore the issues AIDS raises for women, including safer sex, drug-use, pregnancy, lesbians and AIDS, and being antibody positive. Clearly written in an easily accessible style.

Hayman, Suzie, *The Well Woman Handbook* (Penguin, 1989)
Practical and informative, this is an up-to-date guide to the female body, sexually transmitted diseases, contraception and self-help.

USEFUL ADDRESSES

Family Planning Association
27–35 Mortimer Street, London WC1M 7RJ
Tel: 01 636 7866

6 Windsor Place, Cardiff CF1 3BX
Tel: Cardiff 342766

113 University Street, Belfast BT7 1HP
Tel: Belfast 246937

4 Clifton Street, Glasgow G3 7LA
Tel: Glasgow 333 9696

Regional offices which will provide
information on local FPA clinics. Run
through the NHS and you don't need a
GP referral. Provides free and confidential
advice and information on all aspects of
birth control, sexual problems and sexually
transmitted diseases

Irish Family Planning Association
5–7 Cathal Bougha Street, Dublin 2
Tel: Dublin 727276

Provides information on local clinics.
Advice on all aspects of birth control,
women's health, unwanted pregnancies
and sexual problems. Fees according to
how much you earn.

**British Pregnancy Advisory Service
(BPAS)**
Austy Manor, Wooton Wawan, Solihull B95
6BX
Tel: 05642 3225

Clinics in many cities. Confidential and free
pregnancy tests, counselling, advice on

contraception and abortion. Look up in phone book for nearest branch.

Pregnancy Advisory Service (PAS)
13 Charlotte Street, London W1P 1HD
Tel: 01 637 8962

Charity offering information, counselling and practical advice on pregnancy and abortion, contraception, infertility and sexual problems. Fees charged.

Brook Advisory Centres
233 Tottenham Court Road, London W1A 9AE
Tel: 01 580 2991

Provides information on nearest clinic. Gives confidential advice on contraception, pregnancy, abortion and emotional and sexual problems.

Breastcare and Mastectomy Association
26a Harrison Street, London WC1H 8JG
Tel: 01 837 0908

Information and advice on breastcare and mastectomy.

Post-Abortion Counselling Service
340 Westbourne Park Road, London W11 1EQ
Tel: 01 263 7599

Women's Health and Reproductive Rights Information Centre
52 Featherstone Street, London EC1Y 8RT
Tel: 01 251 6580/6332

Information and advice on all aspects of women's health, and reproductive rights and technology.

London Lesbian and Gay Switchboard
BM Switchboard,
London WC1N 3XX
Tel: 01 837 7324

24 hour service. Counselling, help with accommodation and legal affairs. Contact for groups all over Britain.

Relate (Marriage Guidance)
Herbert Gray College, Little Church Street, Rugby CV21 3AP
Tel: 0788 73241

Counselling for problems in all relationships. Can advise on nearest centre.

162

Young People's Counselling Service
Tavistock Centre, 120 Belsize Lane, London
NW3 5BA
Tel: 01 435 7111 (Mon–Fri 9.30 am–5pm)

Free and confidential counselling for young
people from 16–30 who have personal or
emotional problems.

Rape Crisis Centre
PO Box 69, London WC1X 9NJ
Tel: 01 837 1600 (7 days 10am–11pm)

Counselling, medical and legal help on
rape and sexual assault. Look in phone
book for nearest centre or telephone
number.

Chiswick Family Rescue
PO Box 855, London W4 4JF
Tel: 01 995 4430

Provides refuge for women and children
from violence. 24 hour crisis line.

Women's Aid Federation
52–54 Featherstone Street, London EC1Y
8RT
Tel: 01 251 6537

Accommodation and support for women
and children suffering abuse. Groups
throughout England.

Health Education Authority
Hamilton House, Mabledon Place, London
WC1H 9TX
Tel: 01 631 0930

Terrence Higgins Trust
52–54 Gray's Inn Road, London WC1X 8JU
Tel: 01 242 1010/01 833 2971 (helpline)

Advice and counselling for people with
HIV or AIDS and their friends and
relatives. Discussion and support groups
and an information service for those
worried about AIDS.

National AIDS Helpline
Tel: 0800 567123

A free national telephone service with
information and advice on AIDS. They
have a list of AIDS helplines throughout
Britain. Women counsellors are always
available. Afro-Caribbean counsellors Fri
6pm–10pm.

Counselling is also available in the
following languages:

Cantonese, Tues 6pm–10pm 0800 282446

Hindi, Gujerati, Punjabi, Bengali,
Urdu, Wed 6pm–10pm 0800 282445

Healthline Telephone Service
Tel: 0345 581151

24 hour service providing recorded
information on AIDS-related issues.

WALES
Cardiff AIDS Helpline
Tel: Cardiff 2233433 (Mon–Fri 7pm–10pm)

SCOTLAND
Scottish AIDS Monitor
PO Box 169, Edinburgh EH1 3UU
Tel: 031 558 1167 (Mon–Fri 7.30pm–10pm)

Glasgow
Tel: 041 221 7467 (Tues 7pm–10pm)

NORTHERN IRELAND
AIDS Belfast
c/o Cara Friend, PO Box 44, Belfast BT1
1SH
Tel: Belfast 226117 (Mon–Fri
7.30pm–10.30pm)

Blackline
PO Box 74, London SW12 9JY
Tel: 01 727 8384 (Mon–Fri 1pm–4pm)

Helpline, counselling and information
service for Black people who have AIDS.

Positively Women
333 Gray's Inn Road, London WC1X 8PX
Tel: 01 837 9705

A support group for women who are HIV
positive, have ARC or AIDS.

AUSTRALIA

NSW
Family Planning Association of NSW
161 Broadway, Sydney 2007
Tel: 02 211 0244

Help and advice on all aspects of
contraception, sexual problems and sex
education.

Albion Street AIDS Centre
150–154 Albion Street, Surry Hills 2010

Tel: 02 332 4000 (NSW Country callers 008
451 600, TTY number for the hearing
impaired 02 332 4268)

Sydney STD Clinic
Nightingale Centre, Sydney Hospital,
Macquarie Street, Sydney 2000
Tel: 02 247 4851

Rape Crisis Centre
PO Box 188, Drummoyne 2047
Tel: 02 819 6565 (reverse charge 24-hour
service)

Women in Crisis Counselling Service
Wayside Chapel, Hughes Street, Potts
Point 2011
Tel: 02 358 6577

VICTORIA
Family Planning Association of Vic,
266–272 Church Street, Richmond Vic 3121
Tel: 03 429 3500

Women's Information & Referral Exchange
3rd Floor 238 Flinders Lane, Melbourne
3000
Tel: 03 654 6844 (Vic Country callers 008 136
570)

Victoria AIDS Council
61–3 Rupert Street, Collingwood,
Melbourne, Victoria
Tel. 03 417 1759

ACT
Family Planning Association of ACT
Health Promotion Centre, Childers Street,
Canberra ACT 2601
Tel: 062 47 3077

AIDS Information line
Tel. 062 57 2855

QUEENSLAND
Family Planning Association of Qld
100 Alfred Street, Fortitude Valley 4006
Tel: 07 252 5151

Brisbane Women's Health Centre
PO Box 248, Woolloongabba 4102
Tel: 07 844 1935

Information and referral service.

Women's House Rape & Incest Crisis Centre
14 Brook Street, Highgate Hill 4101
Tel: 07 844 4008

24-hour counselling and refuge service.

AIDS Medical Unit
Health & Welfare Building, George Street, Brisbane
Tel: 07 224 5526

Queensland (North) AIDS Council
Tel: 07 844 1990

Queensland (South) AIDS Council
Tel: 07 721 1384

SOUTH AUSTRALIA
Family Planning Association of SA
17 Phillips Street, Kensington SA 5068
Tel: 08 31 5177

AIDS Council of SA
130 Carrington Street, Adelaide 5000
Tel: 08 223 6322

Information and support.

Adelaide Rape Crisis Centre
GPO Box 903, Norwood 5067
Tel: 08 363 0233

Counselling support and advice.

Child, Adolescent & Family Health Service
Tel: 08 236 0400 (SA Country callers 008 188082)

24-hour advisory service.

WESTERN AUSTRALIA
Family Planning Association of WA
70 Roe Street, Northbridge 6000
Tel: 09 227 6177

Western Australia AIDS Council
Tel: 09 227 8355

Women's Health Care House
100 Aberdeen Street, Northbridge 6001
Tel: 09 227 8122

NORTHERN TERRITORY
Family Planning Association of NT
Shop 11, Rapid Creek Shopping Centre, Trower Road, Rapid Creek NT 0810
Tel: 089 480 144

Northern Territory AIDS Council
Tel: 089 41 1711

TASMANIA
Family Planning Association of Tasmania
73 Federal Street, North Hobart Tas 7002
Tel: 002 34 7790

Tasmania AIDS Council
Tel: 002 31 1930

NEW ZEALAND
Family Planning Association
Windsor House, 60 Queen Street, Auckland

2nd Floor, Margaret Sparrow Centre,
45 Tory Street, Wellington

Durham Street Centre, 421 Durham Street,
Christchurch

National Mutual Building, The Octagon,
Dunedin

The AIDS Foundation and AIDS clinics
can be found at:

New Zealand AIDS Foundation,
PO Box 8875, Symonds Street, Auckland

AIDS Clinic
PO Box 6663, Auckland

New Zealand AIDS Foundation
PO Box 7287, Wellington

AIDS Clinic
PO Box 11067, Wellington

AIDS Foundation
NZ AIDS Foundation, PO Box 21285,
Christchurch

New Zealand AIDS Foundation
304 Castle Street, Christchurch

Rape Crisis operates in most centres:

National Rape Crisis
PO Box 6181, Te Aro, Wellington

Rape Crisis Centre
35 Vivian Street, Wellington
Tel: 859 880
62 Ponsonby Road, Ponsonby, Auckland
10 Ventry Street, Alexandra, Otago
PO Box 1327, Hastings
PO Box 673, Palmerston North

PO Box 830, Nelson
Community House, 32 Leach Street, New Plymouth
PO Box 1560, Hamilton
PO Box 368, Tauranga

In Wellington and Auckland two health centres provide services particularly for women:

Otahuhm Medical Centre
115 Church Street, Auckland

Te Aro Health Centre
290 Willis Street, Wellington

CANADA

Barbra Schlifer Commemorative Clinic
490 Adelaide Street West, Suite 201,
Toronto M5V 1T2
Tel: 941 9203

Provides counselling, information, legal advice and a referral service to women who have experienced violence including sexual assault, childhood abuse or rape.

Toronto Counselling Centre for Lesbians and Gays
105 Carlton Street, Top Floor, Toronto M5B 1M2
Tel: 977 2153

Counselling, information and advice.

Inner City Youth Program
Huntley Youth Services, 151 Gerrard Street East, Toronto M5A 2EA
Tel: 922 3335

Counselling and referral on all matters including AIDS.

Planned Parenthood of Toronto
36b Prince Arthur Avenue, Toronto M5R 1A9
Tel: 961 0113

Counselling, referral and medical services for those seeking help on birth control, sexuality and sterilisation.

AIDS Committee of Toronto
Box 55 Station F, Toronto M4Y 2LA
Tel: 926 0063 counselling 926 1626

Grace Hospital Women's Health Centre
1402 8th Avenue, Calgary, Alberta T2R 0G9
Tel: 437 0187

Women's Counselling Services of
Edmonton
145903 10 Avenue, Edmonton, Alberta T5R
5V1
Tel: 483 6320

Vancouver Rape Relief and Women's
Centre
77 E 20th Avenue, Vancouver, BC V5V 1L7
Tel: 872 5212

INDEX

BEING FAT IS NOT A SIN

Shelley Bovey

Being fat is not a sin, but, argues Shelley Bovey, the majority of overweight women are made to feel otherwise.

Pithy and controversial, this book cuts straight to the heart of the fat taboo and uncovers a deep-seated prejudice against fat women. Those who don't fit into society's strict limits on size are not just the butt of seaside postcards; they are considered stupid, incompetent and even deviant.

Shelley Bovey, herself a size 24, exposes discrimination in all its forms, and reveals that this is far more threatening to a woman's physical and mental health than the medical risks associated with being fat. She puts tough questions to Harley St. surgeons, dieticians and others with a vested interest in women wanting to be thinner, and talks to doctors who confess that prejudice, not scientific fact, makes them condemn fat women as 'unhealthy'.

Fat may be a feminist issue but for women who are size 16 and over it is often a miserable reality. Now they share experiences which will strike familiar chords in the heart of every woman who has ever worried about her weight.

Being Fat is Not A Sin helps find a way out of this isolation. It is about losing guilt and inhibition – not about losing weight.

Also Available from Pandora Press

The Hite Report *Shere Hite*	£5.99☐
The Midwife Challenge *Sheila Kitzinger* (ed)	£6.95☐
Drugs in Pregnancy and Childbirth *Judy Priest*	£5.99☐
Miscarriage *Christine Moulder*	£5.99☐
Your Menopause *Myra Hunter*	£5.99☐
Parents' Green Guide *Brigid McConville*	£5.99☐
Being Fat is Not A Sin *Shelley Bovey*	£4.99☐
Living with a Drinker *Mary Wilson*	£4.99☐
Infertility *Renate D Klein* (ed)	£4.95☐
Natural Healing in Gynaecology *Rina Nissim*	£4.95☐
Birth and Our Bodies *Paddy O'Brien*	£4.50☐
Your Life After Birth *Paddy O'Brien*	£4.95☐
Women's Health: A *Spare Rib* Reader *Sue O'Sullivan* (ed)	£5.95☐
The Politics of Breastfeeding *Gabrielle Palmer*	£6.95☐
Motherhood; What It Does To Your Mind *Jane Price*	£4.95☐
Until They Are Five *Angela Phillips*	£4.99☐
Women and the AIDS Crisis *Diane Richardson*	£3.95☐
On Your Own: A Guide to Independent Living *Jean Shapiro*	£6.95☐
The Heroin Users *Tom Stewart*	£5.95☐

All these books are available at your local bookshop or newsagent or can be ordered direct by post.

Just tick the titles you want and fill in the form below.

Name _____

Address _____

_____

Write to Unwin Hyman Cash Sales, PO Box 11, Falmouth, Cornwall TR10 9ED.
Please enclose remittance to the value of the cover price plus:
UK: 80p for the first book plus 20p for each additional book ordered to a maximum charge of £2.00.

BFPO: 80p for the first book plus 20p for each additional book.

OVERSEAS INCLUDING EIRE: £1.50 for the first book plus £1 for each additional book.

Unwin Hyman Paperbacks reserve the right to show new retail prices on covers, which may differ from those previously advertised in the text or elsewhere. Postage rates are subject to revision.